Reflections on Health

Commemorating Fifty Years
of
The Department of Health
1947–1997

Editor:
Joseph Robins

First Published in 1997
by the
Department of Health
Dublin
Ireland

i 14032430

British Library Cataloguing in Publication Data
A catalogue record for this book is available from the British Library.

ISBN 1 872002 39 0

Publishing Consultants: Institute of Public Administration

Cover design by Butler Claffey, Dun Laoghaire
Typeset by Alan Hodgson
Printed by Smurfit Print, Dublin

Contents

Foreword

Brian Cowen TD, Minister for Health and Children

Many changes for the better have taken place in this country in the past fifty years. Not the least of these is the transformation in the health of the Irish people. In the 1940s children died in their thousands from preventable diseases, many young adults wasted from tuberculosis, mothers died unnecessarily in child birth and the health of the public was constantly threatened by outbreaks of typhoid, typhus and polio. A healthy old age was the privilege of a minority.

It was public concern at the unacceptable toll of mortality and morbidity that led in 1947 to the appointment of a Minister for Health, Dr Jim Ryan, and the creation of a separate department. The new minister and department lost no time in putting health at the centre of the government's agenda. Since that time, the combined efforts of politicians, health professionals and public servants have translated advances in medicine, science and technology into services that have given Irish people one of the highest standards of health in the world.

The challenge facing the health services in the new millennium may be different but, as the articles in this book make clear, no less daunting than that facing our predecessors fifty years ago. Too many of our contemporaries die unnecessarily from heart disease, cancer and accidents. Our success in raising life expectancy means that many more older people will depend on the health services to keep them going. We have a long road to travel before we can say that all our children have an equal opportunity for health. The development of science and technology are raising the most profound ethical issues for society and the health services in particular. And we must make sure that, as far as humanly possible, no health service is ever again the cause of ill-health and suffering such as that experienced by those infected through the anti-D product.

As Minister for Health and Children, on the threshold of the new century, I look forward to carrying on the good work of my predecessors and to contributing, in partnership with all those associated with the health services, towards the resolution of many of the issues raised in this important book.

The Contributors

EDITOR

JOSEPH ROBINS, B.COMM., DIP.PUB.AD., PH.D., F.INST.HOSP.ADMIN., is a former assistant secretary of the Department of Health. He is currently actively involved with a number of bodies in the voluntary sector. A social historian, his books include *The Lost Children* (a history of Irish charity children), *Fools and Mad* (a history of insanity in Ireland), *From Rejection to Integration* (the growth of services for persons with mental handicap) and *The Miasma* (epidemic and public health in 19th century Ireland).

CONTRIBUTORS

MICHAEL BOLAND, M.I.C.G.P., F.R.C.G.P., is Director, Postgraduate Resource Centre, Irish College of General Practitioners.

PATRICIA BROWN, B.SOC.SC., M.SOC.SC., is a senior research officer in the Institute of Public Administration, Dublin, and a lecturer on the Institute's post graduate programme in public management. She is working on a research based PH.D. with Brunel University.

GEOFFREY CHADWICK, B.SC., M.B., B.C.H., B.A.O., M.D., F.R.C.P.I., is Director of the Centre for Medical Education at University College Dublin and Dun's Tutor (postgraduate co-ordinator) at the Royal College of Physicians of Ireland. He is a practising physician with a special interest in medical education.

DAVIS COAKLEY, M.D., F.R.C.P.I., F.R.C.P. (LONDON), is Professor of Medical Gerontology at Trinity College Dublin and Consultant Physician, Department of Medicine for the Elderly, St James's Hospital Dublin.

ANNE COLGAN, B.A., M.ED., is an independent consultant in organisational development, evaluation and training in the health and educational fields. She was formerly Manager, Youth Employment and Advisory Service and Manager Research and Planning with the National Rehabilitation Board.

SEAN CONROY, B.SC., H.DIP.ED., M.B., B.CH., B.A.O., L.M.C.C., is Programme Manager, General Hospital Care with the Western Health Board.

DENIS CUSACK, F.R.C.P.I., B.L., is Director of the Division of Legal Medicine, University College Dublin. He is a specialist in legal and forensic medicine and founder editor of the *Medico-Legal Journal of Ireland.*

JOHN DEVLIN, M.B., B.SC., D.C.H., M.P.H., F.F.P.H.M.I., F.R.C.P.I., is Deputy Chief Medical Officer of the Department of Health.

PAULINE FAUGHNAN, M.SOC.SC., PH.D., is Senior Research Fellow and EU Research Co-Ordinator at the Social Science Research Centre, University College Dublin. She worked for some time in the voluntary sector and continues to be involved in that area.

OWEN KEENAN, B.SOC.SC., C.C.E.T.S.W., DIP.S.W., CERT.PUB.AD., is Director-General of Barnardo's (Rep. of Ireland) and current President of the European Forum for Child Welfare.

C. CECILY KELLEHER, M.D., F.R.C.P.I., M.P.H., F.F.P.H.M., M.F.P.H.M.I., has been Professor of Health Promotion at University College Galway since 1990. She is also a director of two research centres associated with the College: the Centre for Health Promotion Studies and the National Nutritional Surveillance Centre.

GERALDINE McCARTHY, R.G.N., R.N.T., M.ED., M.S.N., PH.D., is Director of the Department of Nursing Studies at University College Cork. She was formerly Nursing Research and Development Manager at Beaumont Hospital Dublin.

EVELYN MAHON, B.A., M.A., M.SC. (ECON.), is a lecturer in the Department of Sociology and Director of the Women and Pregnancy Study at Trinity College Dublin. She has written on the women's movement and on gender equality and is working on a PH.D. with London University.

JERRY O'DWYER, B.A., is Secretary of the Department of Health.

HAROLD O'SULLIVAN, M.LITT., PH.D., Honorary Fellow Environmental Health Officers Association, is former General Secretary of the Irish Local Government and Public Services Union and a past President of the Irish Congress of Trade Unions.

BRION SWEENEY, M.B., B.CH., B.A.O., D.C.H., M.MED.SC. (PSYCHOTHERAPY), M.R.C.PSYCH., is Consultant Psychiatrist in Substance Misuse with the Eastern Health Board Addictions Services.

DERMOT WALSH, F.R.C.P.I., is Inspector of Mental Hospitals, Department of Health; Clinical Director, St. Loman's Hospital, Dublin; has responsibilities for the Mental Health Section, Health Research Board, Dublin.

MIRIAM M. WILEY, M.SC., PH.D., is Head of the Health Policy Research Centre and Senior Research Officer at the Economic and Social Research Institute, Dublin. She has published extensively on health care financing, reform, management, organisation and delivery.

CHAPTER 1

Introduction

Joseph Robins

From their individual professional perspectives the distinguished contributors to this book have viewed critically the progress of Irish health and its supporting services over the last fifty years. What emerges is a chronicle of remarkable advance.

Looked at in the simplest terms, the changes in the pattern of health during the period surveyed are striking. Reductions in mortality generally have given rise to increased life expectancy at birth from 61 to 73 years for males and from 62 to 79 years for females. The infant mortality rate has fallen from 68 per 1000 births in 1947 to six at present. Maternal mortality can now be described as a rare event. In the light of these figures it will be difficult for many to understand the thinking that, at the beginning of the period under review, forced a Minister for Health from office because he sought to make maternity and child health services more widely available.

But the quality of our national health and of the services maintaining it must be judged in wider terms than those of the statistics of mortality. There are other important considerations. They include the caring philosophy on which the services are based, their availability and range, the equality of all seeking care, the degree of sensitivity to the human condition and particularly the acceptance that good health is more than the absence of illness, it is a general state of wellbeing.

The contributions that follow indicate significant progress in all these areas. Underlying the changes has been the increasing emphasis given to human dignity and individuality. Indeed if the period 1947-1997 had made no contribution to the advancement of the practice of humanity but the recognition of the dignity and rights of the disadvantaged individual, it would have been an outstanding one. Fifty years ago many thousands of citizens with mental illness or mental handicap, elderly and infirm persons in need of care, unwanted and deprived children, outcast unmarried mothers, were being cared for en masse in large institutions of mainly nineteenth century origin. Patients of little means needing basic medical care were subjected to the discriminating and restrictive requirements of the Victorian dispensary doctor system. Those of modest means requiring hospital treatment received no support from the state and often had to face intolerable financial burdens. Persons who were functionally, economically and socially disadvantaged by longterm disability were ignored, written off by society, with little effort made to integrate or reintegrate them in normal living activity. Our modern health services show radical change in all these areas.

Other changes have led to greater geographic equity. The development of regional hospitals and the upgrading of selected county hospitals have brought many specialist services closer to provincial areas, and represent an enormous advance on the former one-surgeon, one-physician county hospital.

Ironically, at a time when the traditional family unit is being eroded, society has come to recognise that the ideal environment for the therapy and care of the individual is the setting of the family and the community of families. If, however, the longterm institution has a much lesser role than in the past, the importance and potential of the acute hospital for the investigation and therapy of illness has grown. There have been remarkable scientific and technological advances in chemotherapy, surgical procedures, investigative medicine, psychotherapy and prevention which have contributed enormously to the reduction of suffering and mortality. More than any other area of the health services, the complexity and cost of the modern acute hospital reflects the advance of twentieth century medicine. In 1947 the total cost to the state of *all* health services was less than £6 million: today it is about £2.5 billion, of which approximately half goes towards the operation of the public general hospital services.

WHERE DO WE GO FROM HERE?

In important respects we now have greater control over disease than we had fifty years ago. Large-scale infectious disease is, for example, no longer a problem, although AIDS remains a threat. But the control of the two major causes of mortality – cardiovascular disease and cancer – is to an important degree a matter for the individual since these conditions may arise from one's chosen life style. While the main thrust of the health services will continue to be in the area of providing for sickness, the greatest potential for further improvement in the pattern of our national health lies in policies directed at health promotion and the prevention of ill-health in the first instance. This is not a matter for the health services exclusively. It necessarily requires the conscious participation of all socio-economic elements influencing the life-style of the individual so that policies, practices and attitudes are formed with a consciousness of their likely impact on the health of the citizen.

It is clear from the contributions to this book that there are still significant health inequalities in our society and that their reduction must be an essential component of health promotion policy. The children of families at risk due to deprivation, parental inadequacy or family breakdown are more likely during their lifespan to require the involvement of health and other social services, and to become lesser citizens as adults, because the odds were stacked against them in childhood. Clearly there will be a continuing need for additional resources for the support of families at risk. The vulnerability of young people to drug hazards must remain a priority of public concern. The special health hazards of women require greater recognition. The extent of violence against women and the need for rape crisis centres and women's aid havens are a shame on twentieth century society. Another shame is the continuing marginalisation of the small travelling community, reflected in particular in its unfavourable statistics of morbidity and mortality.

Even allowing for the beneficial longterm influences of the growth of a cultural environment of health promotion, it is likely that the cost of health services will go on increasing inexorably. We have now reached the point where public expenditure on health represents over 20% of all public expenditure and approximately 6.5% of gross national product. Past expansions in services and the perennial increase of public expenditure in the health area have not always been accompanied by a sufficient questioning of the efficiency of the administrative organisations and procedures involved. Management of, and within, the health services has become a major priority of public policy, not only to seek optimum value from the huge commitment of resources but because the quality of health care itself may be influenced by the quality of management.

There are many management issues to be confronted in both broad and narrow areas. Health boards are not forever. They have been a stage in the continuing evolution of local administrations. Apart from the huge expansion in the range, technology and cost of services since the boards were established, the movement towards greater devolution of central authority must have an impact on their present structures. There is a need to give service users and service providers a greater involvement in the decision-making process. Furthermore it is important to recognise that the concept of health as a state of general wellbeing implies that responsibility for it lies not entirely, or even largely, within the narrow medical domain. Social workers, for instance, are having wider demands made on their skills. The nursing profession, inclined traditionally to be unobtrusive, has a case for a greater role

7

in management and decision making. Greater recognition should be accorded to the voluntary area, not merely to using it, but to strengthening its considerable contribution and clearly involving it in the various levels of policy and decision making.

For most members of the public the first point of contact with the health system is the family doctor. The skills and professional relationships of general practice within the system must be further developed and more clearly defined.

There are many issues to be confronted in the hospital services. They include the governance of hospitals, the creation of quality management systems within them, the identification from the consumer's viewpoint of the most beneficial arrangements for the mix of public and private practice, and the need for clearer understandings about the participation in management of the medical consultants. A desirable aim should be the retention of strong corporate and professional cultures in the voluntary hospitals while delivering services within a national policy framework.

Future public issues and controversies in the health area are increasingly more likely to be concerned with medico-legal and ethical problems than with relatively uncomplicated issues such as shortages of finance or the location of services. Contemporary society has created its own philosophical climate. There is a greater sensitivity to what are perceived to be individual 'rights', a questioning of some long-established and previously sacrosanct human values, the potential of medical science to influence or manipulate human biology in ways previously regarded as fantasy. The issues are already there but are likely to grow in intensity. Genetic engineering, infertility, in-vitro fertilisation, amniocentesis, abortion, sterilisation, euthanasia and other as yet unidentified areas are likely to raise profound questions not only for the professionals involved but for government and for the individual in twenty-first century society.

I feel honoured by the Department of Health to be asked to edit this collection of essays to mark the fiftieth anniversary of its establishment. I would emphasise that the record of progress described by the contributors is not intended as a paean to the Department; it should be seen as a tribute to all those involved in the advance of our health over the last half century, the politicians and administrators, the professionals and others in the caring area or in supporting scientific and technical roles, whether in statutory bodies, religious or voluntary organisations or in a private capacity. The progress recorded is the total outcome of all their contributions.

We face the health challenges of a new century from a position of considerable strength.

The concept of this book received the full support of Michael Noonan TD, as Minister for Health and the Secretary of the Department, Jerry O'Dwyer. I thank Ruth Barrington for her part in working out the concept of this book and in advancing its publication. I am grateful to all the contributors for making it possible. I would like to acknowledge the assistance of Adrienne Brunty in helping me to assemble it. I thank Helen Litton for her editing skills and I am grateful to Tony McNamara and his colleagues in the publications division of the Institute of Public Administration for their advice and their expertise.

Joseph Robins
Editor
July 1997

CHAPTER 2

The State of Health in Ireland

John Devlin

INTRODUCTION

Health is not easy to define. For some people, health conveys an absence of disease, but this lacks a positive description of what is meant by health. The World Health Organisation defines health as – 'a state of complete physical, mental and social well-being, not merely the absence of disease or infirmity' *(Constitution of the World Health Organisation: Basic Documents 15th Edition, Geneva 1961)*. This might be considered Utopian but, while few people would consider themselves as completely healthy using such criteria, it does offer a definition which is useful from the viewpoint of therapeutic goals and the effectiveness of health services. Health may be regarded as the optimal adaptation of an individual to his/her physical, psychological and social environment. It is difficult to measure and over the years a number of health status indicators have been developed to act as a proxy for measurement of health. These indicators have proved useful in monitoring progress towards health-related targets and include life expectancy, mortality and morbidity information, lifestyle, and environmental health data and information on the healthcare system.

Health status may be influenced by a number of factors including lifestyle, environmental and occupational hazards, and genetic inheritance of certain conditions. In the nineteenth and early twentieth centuries, major health problems were primarily associated with under-nutrition, crowding, exhaustion and inadequate water supplies. These conditions resulted in a high prevalence of tuberculosis, gastro-enteritis, respiratory diseases and high infant mortality. In response, improved economic and social conditions together with public health action have virtually eliminated the pandemics of infectious disease. The decline of the traditional infectious diseases has been mastered largely through the provision of safe drinking water, effective vaccine campaigns, improved personal hygiene and better nutrition, especially among children. While many of these infectious diseases have been controlled, others have taken their place, and the emergence of AIDS world-wide underscores the fact that infectious diseases are likely to remain an important problem, even in developed countries, for many years to come.

With regard to environmental hazards, the major concern of the twentieth century has been the provision of biologically safe water and food to the population, and the safe removal of sewage and rubbish. While systems are now in place to undertake these functions, exposure to chemicals and radiation is a continuing problem and requires careful monitoring. Unfortunately, some of the health effects from such pollution may occur years after exposure and are therefore difficult to evaluate. Safeguarding the health of workers and the general population from environmental hazards will present an ongoing challenge for the years to come.

As we approach the end of the twentieth century, developed countries are facing major health problems in the form of chronic diseases which are often related to lifestyle, namely diet, smoking and excessive alcohol consumption. Heart disease and cancer are the leading causes of premature mortality today. Life expectancy in Ireland has increased significantly over the past fifty years and, until recently, this was due to the reduction of fatal diseases in infancy and the early years of life. Today the decrease in mortality during the later years of life has become the major factor in influencing life expectancy, and it will likely prove difficult to emulate the progress seen in the past fifty years. The challenges in preventing and controlling chronic disease relate not only to extending the duration of life but also to maintaining the quality of that extended life. As in other developed countries, Ireland's population is ageing, and this will present new challenges to the health and social services over the coming decades. As people live longer, they are more likely to develop a disabling illness which may restrict their activity and require therapeutic intervention. Heart disease and arthritis have been identified as common conditions which may result in substantial limitation of activity.

Healthcare policy in Europe has undergone significant change over the course of the twentieth century. Initial priorities were concerned with provision of access to physicians and this was followed by priority for hospital development. After this phase, other areas were afforded greater priority, such as mental health and care for the elderly. This was followed by the promotion of comprehensive integrated healthcare systems and the development of healthcare personnel as the crucial resource. In recent years, the emphasis has been on more efficient healthcare, cost containment and the equitable distribution of available resources. Since 1947, when the Department of Health was established, very good progress has been made in improving the health of our population as a whole. The Department of Health's strategy for effective healthcare (*Shaping a Healthier Future*, Department of Health, Dublin 1994) was concerned with the reorientation of the Irish healthcare system by reshaping the way services were planned and delivered. Efficient use of resources, equitably distributed, together with a high quality of service were considered key factors in maximising health and social gain for the years to come. Targets have been set with regard to Irish life expectancy and premature mortality which are directly relevant to future generations.

This chapter reviews the health status of Irish people in 1947, traces developments to the present day and makes comparisons within the European context. Health status indicators which include life expectancy, mortality and demographic data form the basis of these comparisons. Finally, this chapter speculates on future influences on health status and the likely challenges to the provision of health services in the years to come.

AS IT WAS IN 1947

Vital Statistics reports which are published annually provide information on births, marriages and deaths over the past 50 years. The report of the Registrar General for 1947 contains detailed information on births, marriages and deaths similar to that which is collected today (*Annual Report of the Registrar General 1947*, Department of Health, Dublin 1949). Whilst the definitions of particular diseases may have changed somewhat over the years, it is possible nevertheless to make valid comparisons between the health of the nation as it was in 1947 and today. A snapshot of health and social status for the year 1947 as described by the Registrar General is provided below.

MARRIAGES AND BIRTHS

Registered marriages during 1947 numbered 16,290 which gave a rate of 5.5 per 1,000 population, and it is interesting that this rate was lower than Northern Ireland, Scotland, England and Wales.

Births in 1947 numbered 68,978, a figure which was 7,600 more than the average number recorded for the previous ten years. This gave a rate of 23.2 per 1,000 population which was similar to Northern Ireland, but greater than Scotland, England and Wales. Information on births outside marriage revealed that in 1947 there were 2,348 such births which represented 3.4% of the total births recorded. This figure was less than the rates recorded in Northern Ireland, Scotland, England and Wales. The vast majority of live births (98.6%) involved mothers giving birth to single infants.

12

DEMOGRAPHY

Information on the structure of Ireland's population has been collected by census at approximately five yearly intervals throughout this century. In 1946, the population of Ireland at 2.96 million was close to its nadir in recent times. This contrasted to a population of over 6.5 million approximately 100 years previously (Census of Population of Ireland, Central Statistics Office, Dublin, Reports 1946-1996) (Figure 1).

FIGURE 1

Population of Ireland 1841-1996

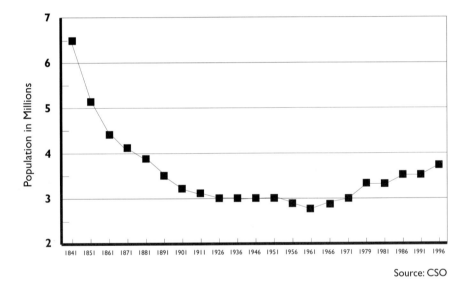

Source: CSO

The dramatic decline in Ireland's population between 1841 and 1946 was not evenly distributed across the country. The population of Leinster fell slightly from 1.97 million to 1.28 million whereas, in contrast, the population of Munster fell from 2.4 million to 0.92 million, Connaught from 1.42 million to half a million and Ulster from 740,000 to 264,000 people.

MORTALITY

In 1947 there were 44,061 deaths which gave a rate of 14.8 per 1,000 population. The death rate at this time remained relatively constant but represented considerable improvement from the late nineteenth century when it was approximately 18 per 1,000 population. It was interesting that more than 5,500 deaths (12.5% of the total) were not stated to have been certified by a medical practitioner or coroner. The major causes of death in 1947 are shown in Figure 2.

FIGURE 2

Principal Causes of Death 1947

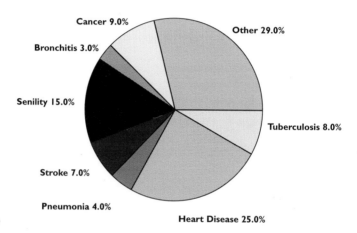

Source: CSO

There are significant differences between mortality in 1947 and today (Figure 9). In 1947 the major causes of death included heart disease, 'senility' and infectious diseases including tuberculosis. This is in marked contrast to the major causes of mortality today, which include cardiovascular disease and cancer. In 1947, there was considerable mortality from infectious diseases which included not only tuberculosis but also conditions such as typhoid fever, scarlet fever, whooping cough, diphtheria, influenza, polio, and measles.

Infant mortality in 1947 was 68 per 1,000 births and had changed little over the preceding decade. This rate was higher than that recorded in Northern Ireland, Scotland, England and Wales for that period. The major causes of infant mortality were prematurity (12%), congenital debility (11%), gastro-enteritis (10%) and pneumonia (9%). In children aged between one and five years, the vast majority of deaths were caused by infectious diseases including pneumonia, tuberculosis, whooping cough, measles, gastro-enteritis and diphtheria. In older children aged between five and fifteen years, the most common cause of death was tuberculosis. Tuberculosis was also the major cause of death amongst adolescents and young adults under forty-five years of age.

1947 TO PRESENT DAY

BIRTHS AND MARRIAGES

Over the past fifty years, the marriage rate generally increased and peaked in the 1970s but has been declining since then (Figure 3). The average age at marriage was falling until 1984; however it has increased since and the most recent census analysis showed that the average age for males was 28.7 years and for females 26.9 years (*Report on Vital Statistics, 1991,* Central Statistics Office, Dublin 1996). Most households today are composed of single family units, followed by one-person households and other categories. For many years, there has been a trend towards smaller household size (the number of persons in the household).

During the past fifty years, there have been significant changes regarding the number of registered births in Ireland. In the 1940s, there were approximately 65,000 births per annum and this number slowly increased and peaked in 1980 at 74,000 births. Since then there has been a rapid decline and in 1995 approximately 48,500 births were recorded. The corresponding birth rates are shown in Figure 3.

FIGURE 3

Births, Deaths & Marriages

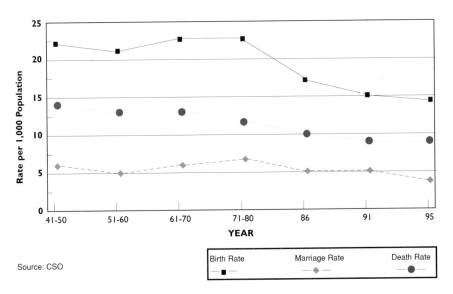

Source: CSO

The average age at maternity has risen in recent years and now stands at 29.3 years. A significant change has taken place with regard to the numbers of births outside marriage, increasing rapidly from 2% of births in the 1950s to 22% today.

DEMOGRAPHY

Since 1961, Ireland's population has been increasing, albeit slowly, and in 1996 stood at slightly over 3.6 million. This increase has been mainly in Leinster and to a lesser degree in Munster and Connaught, whereas in Ulster the population has actually declined.

The age distribution of Ireland's population has changed remarkably little in the past fifty years (Figure 4). Overall, the population has become a little older. About 40% of the population are in the 'dependent' category, that is, they are either younger than fourteen or older than sixty-five years of age.

The age structure of Ireland's population in 1994 is in marked contrast to the

FIGURE 4

Ireland's Population

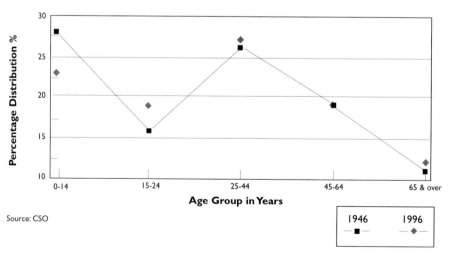

Source: CSO

	1946	1996
	—■—	—◆—

European Union's average, which is more mature with relatively few children compared to Ireland (*Demographic Statistics 1995,* Eurostat, Statistical Office of the European Communities, Luxembourg 1995) (Figure 5).

FIGURE 5

Population by Age Group

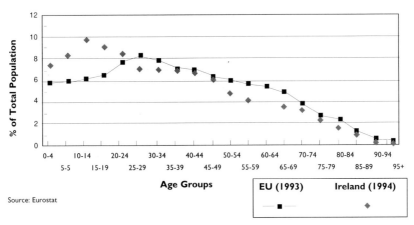

Age Groups

Source: Eurostat

| EU (1993) | Ireland (1994) |

The changes in Ireland's population over the past fifty years represent the balance between the natural increase (excess of births over deaths) and the net migration of the population. The decline in emigration has contributed towards population growth in recent years.

POPULATION PROJECTIONS

Population projections have been made for Ireland from 1996 up to the year 2026 (*Population and Labour Force Projections 1996-2026*, Central Statistics Office, Dublin 1995). These projections are based on assumptions regarding Irish fertility patterns, mortality and migration. The net result is a significant change in the population structure for Ireland in the years to come (Figure 6).

FIGURE 6

Population Projection for Ireland

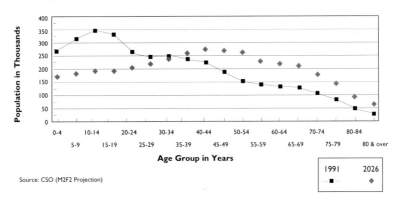

Age Group in Years

Source: CSO (M2F2 Projection)

| 1991 | 2026 |

The population structure will adopt the shape of a mature population, similar to that of many European countries today. The major changes which emerge are the expansions in the middle and old age groups, together with a contraction in the younger age groups. The total dependency ratio is projected to decline until approximately the year 2006 and then increase again, primarily as a result of the increase in the elderly population. The increase in the older population (age sixty-five years and older) will be particularly striking in the period 2006-2026. The population for this age group is projected to increase to almost 700,000 people by the year 2026. This represents almost a doubling of the population aged over sixty-five years and the increase will be most marked in the very old population (i.e. greater than eighty years of age). These changes are primarily due to the improvements in life expectancy which are likely in the coming years.

DEATHS

Over the past fifty years, the number of deaths in Ireland has been slowly decreasing. In the 1940s the average number of deaths per annum was approximately 42,000 and this has fallen by 10,000 today. This is reflected in the death rate which in the 1940s was fourteen and today is less than nine (Figure 3). This mortality reduction has increased life expectancy (Figure 7). Fifty years ago, life expectancy at birth of males and females was sixty-one and sixty-two years respectively, today it is approximately seventy-three and seventy-eight years.

FIGURE 7

Life Expectancy at Birth

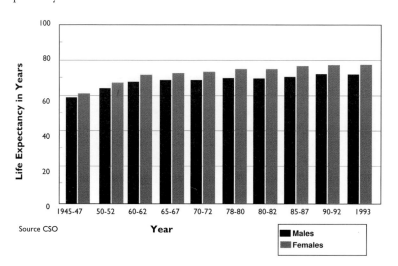

Source CSO

Males
Females

Major changes in the pattern of mortality have been seen over the past fifty years. Mortality from infectious diseases, including tuberculosis (Figure 8), influenza and measles, has dropped dramatically and they no longer feature amongst the most important causes of death. While mortality from the 'traditional' infectious diseases has reduced, the emergence of Human Immunodeficiency Virus (HIV) and AIDS has partially countered this trend. Up to the end of 1996 there were 1,731 cases of HIV, 577 AIDS cases and 304 deaths due to AIDS. Intravenous drug use accounted for the largest single category (43%) of AIDS cases in Ireland; this contrasts with the European experience where AIDS is predominantly a sexually transmitted disease.

FIGURE 8

Respiratory Tuberculosis Mortality

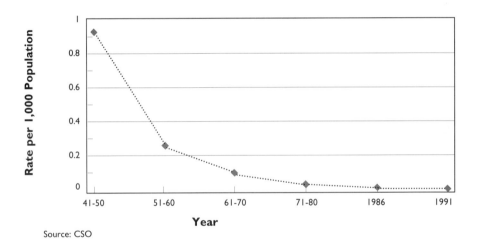

Source: CSO

Cardiovascular disease, which includes coronary heart disease and stroke, continues to be one of the most important causes of death and today accounts for two out of every five deaths in Ireland. The death rate from cancer has been slowly increasing and now causes one in four deaths every year. Deaths due to 'senility' have reduced dramatically, predominantly due to changes in coding practice over the intervening years. The principal causes of death are shown in Figure 9.

FIGURE 9

Principal Causes of Death 1995

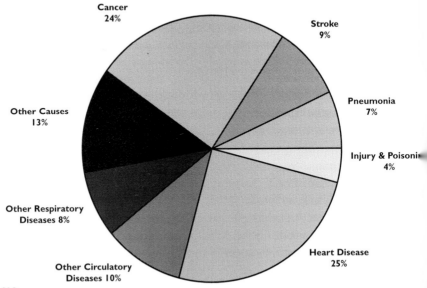

Cancer
24%

Stroke
9%

Other Causes
13%

Pneumonia
7%

Injury & Poisoni⯑
4%

Other Respiratory
Diseases 8%

Heart Disease
25%

Other Circulatory
Diseases 10%

Source: CSO

MATERNAL AND INFANT MORTALITY

Maternal mortality has fallen dramatically over the years and today there are only two or three deaths every year. There have also been large decreases in infant and neo-natal mortality during this time (Figure 10).

FIGURE 10

Infant Neonatal Mortality Rates

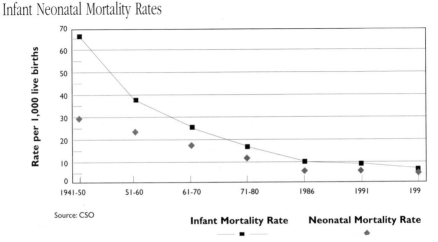

Source: CSO

Infant Mortality Rate

Neonatal Mortality Rate

The major cause of infant mortality today is due to congenital abnormalities (44%); infections have become much less significant in recent years and now account for less than 5% of infant mortality.

HEALTH POLICY AND HEALTH

Ireland's health status in 1947, with a life expectancy of approximately 60 years, significant mortality from infectious diseases and the high infant death rate, was important in determining priorities for the Department of Health in the early years. The Tuberculosis Act 1945, which enabled the building of hospitals for the care of patients with tuberculosis, together with the Health Act 1947 which provided for free treatment, improved social support and vaccination, both had a significant impact on this major disease. With regard to preventive services in the areas of infectious diseases and food hygiene, the Health Act 1947 modernised the original Public Health (Ireland) Act 1878 and provided for free hospital treatment for infectious diseases. Within a few years, mortality from tuberculosis and other infectious diseases was greatly reduced.

Other priority areas at that time included the extension of hospital services to cover most of the population, improving eligibility for general practitioner services, the development of child welfare clinicals and school health services. The Health Act 1953 was a significant landmark, allowing for the broader provision of hospital services, and this, together with the post-war building programme of new hospitals and the sanctioning of additional consultant appointments, greatly improved access to hospital services. The Act also extended maternity and child care services. These changes had the general effect of greatly improving the standard of hospital and preventive services and during the following decade, Ireland experienced one of its largest increases in life expectancy ever seen in recent times.

The following years were a period of consolidation of the health services and, as priorities changed, so did the evaluation and planning of services to meet new health needs. Within a few short years, infant mortality and infectious diseases, including tuberculosis, had become less significant and in their place emerged diseases associated with ageing including heart disease and cancer. It was also realised that to take advantage of improvements in healthcare and new technology, it was necessary to introduce new administrative arrangements to maximise access to healthcare. The Health Act 1970 introduced many new changes for primary healthcare, including improved access to general practitioners via the choice of doctor scheme, and the establishment of the home help service. Health Boards were established and these had responsibility for the provision of healthcare services within

21

their regions. In this period several bodies were established which advised the Department of Health on special issues, for example the National Drugs Advisory Board, the Health Education Bureau and Comhairle na nOspidéal. These agencies proved to be an invaluable resource and facilitated the Department of Health in its general planning, organisation and delivery of effective healthcare services.

It is not always easy to link policy developments with immediate changes in health status. These effects are most demonstrable in community protection programmes. In recent years, further advances have been made regarding control of certain infectious diseases, for example measles and haemophilus meningitis, by immunisation schemes. It has proved more difficult to modify lifestyle. However, progress has been made on reducing smoking by regulating the promotion of tobacco products and by health education. This has contributed significantly towards the reduction in premature mortality from lung cancer in men that has been observed in recent years. The recent health strategy, *Shaping a Healthier Future*, places an onus on those who plan and deliver health services to reflect the principles of equity, quality of service and accountability in the development of services so as to maximise health and social gain in future years.

IRELAND'S PLACE IN EUROPE

HEALTH IN EUROPE

During the nineteenth and early twentieth centuries, Europe experienced great advances in public health, primarily from the realisation that unsatisfactory water supplies, sanitation, working conditions, food, housing and air were major contributors to disease and short life-spans. These advances have continued in recent times and most European countries have demonstrated increased life expectancy. The elimination of some infectious diseases, reduced mortality from many of the leading causes of death, and reduced infant and maternal mortality has contributed towards these advances. As infectious diseases contributed less to overall mortality in recent years, the focus is turning to what are now the two major causes of mortality, namely cardiovascular disease and cancer. Lifestyle is recognised as an important risk factor for these diseases and throughout Europe, health promotion related activities have become increasingly important. Progress in promoting lifestyles conducive to health has however been moderate. Overall, the growing trend towards non-smoking has been the most noticeable factor in recent years.

Another area of major concern is the lack of progress towards achieving the primary target, namely equity in health, of the World Health Organisation's Health for All by 2000 Programme (*Health For All Targets; The Health Policy for Europe,* Updated Edition, World Health Organisation, Copenhagen, 1991). There is evidence of a widening gap in health status, not only between countries in Europe but also between groups within countries. Many European countries also share common problems including an ageing population, increasing costs of health and social services and generally slow progress in health promotion and many preventive services. Healthcare reforms have been initiated in many countries but progress towards high quality and efficient care is far from what it could be. These problems, together with the issue of equity in health, are the major challenges facing Europe for the coming decades.

In comparison with many European countries, Ireland has built its recent health policy on the WHO's Health for All by 2000 Programme. The primary aim is to enhance the health and quality of life of people. Health and social gain are central aspects of the Irish health strategy. While it is difficult to measure social gain, health gain is measurable by increases in life expectancy and a reduction in premature mortality. Information on these indicators is also available at European level, and comparisons are provided below.

LIFE EXPECTANCY

A welcome increase in Irish life expectancy has been observed over the past fifty years and for males is similar to the European Union average; however, female life expectancy in Ireland is less than European levels. The large increase in life expectancy at birth in Ireland was due primarily to a reduction in infant and childhood mortality. In contrast only modest increases have been seen in life expectancy for the middle-aged and elderly Irish population, and our life expectancy at these ages is below the European Union average. Premature mortality from cardiovascular disease and cancer has hindered progress towards improved life expectancy in middle and old age in Ireland.

PREMATURE MORTALITY

Approximately one-fifth of all deaths in Ireland are in people aged less than sixty-five years of age. Cancer, cardiovascular disease and accidents account for the majority of these deaths and much of this mortality is preventable. In recent years, mortality from coronary heart disease has fallen in Ireland, but it remains above the European Union average (Figure 11).

FIGURE 11

Premature Mortality

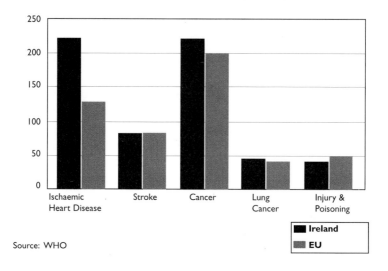

Source: WHO

It is encouraging that the death rate from stroke has fallen dramatically in recent years and is now similar to the EU average. While the overall death rate from cancer is rising and is above the European Union average, a welcome reduction in cancer mortality has been observed in the under sixty-fives in recent years. Lung cancer mortality has fallen recently but remains above the EU average. In spite of a recent increase in road traffic accident mortality in the past year, the general trend is towards a reduced mortality from this cause and Irish rates are similar to those in Europe. It is encouraging that mortality from accidents in general has fallen significantly in recent years and is well below European levels. Ireland's improvement with regard to infant mortality in recent years means that it now has one of the lowest rates within Europe.

CHALLENGES FOR THE FUTURE

MEETING THE CHALLENGE : THE HEALTH STRATEGY

Health is widely regarded as the corner-stone of the wealth of a nation. Health and well-being are inextricably linked to the overall condition of life. The primary aim of the Department of Health and the health services is to enhance the health and quality of life of people. Health is a determinant of and a contributor to the general economic and social development of all countries.

Poor health in the population limits the country's effectiveness in achieving desirable standards of productivity and efficiency and likewise, poor economic conditions limit the development of adequate health and social services.

The Irish health strategy, *Shaping a Healthier Future*, is focused on increasing the health and social gain of Irish people. The strategy recommends the reorientation of the healthcare system in terms of how services are planned and delivered so that health and social gain will be maximised. These aims may be measured by increases in life expectancy, reductions in morbidity and mortality and also by improvements in the general quality of life. The strategy is underpinned by the key principles of equity, quality of service and accountability. If the overall aims of the strategy are to be achieved, access to healthcare should be determined by actual need, health services must meet the highest possible quality standards and healthcare providers must be responsible for the achievement of agreed objectives. The strategy has set targets with regard to improving life expectancy and reducing premature mortality amongst Irish people. The major causes of premature mortality were highlighted and specific objectives were set in relation to reducing mortality from cancer, cardiovascular disease and accidents. Improvements in these areas, together with the elimination of health inequalities across the population, will have a significant impact on the health status of Irish people in the coming years.

HEALTH PROMOTION

In recent years the experience in developed countries is that higher standards of living offer greater choices of lifestyle including health-damaging behaviour. In Ireland, smoking has been identified as one of the major risk factors causing premature mortality and the recent reduction in smoking prevalence must be maintained if such premature mortality is to be avoided. Improving information and giving people more control over their living and working environments should enable people to make healthier choices, and therefore improve the quality of life and increase the level of health in the population.

ENVIRONMENTAL CONCERNS

Unsatisfactory environmental conditions played an important part in adversely affecting health in the nineteenth and early twentieth centuries. While significant improvements have been achieved, it is important to evaluate potential environmental hazards because of their threat to health. Water and air quality, food safety, waste management and air pollution together with hazards in the work environment require careful monitoring. It is sometimes difficult to evaluate the risk to health and it may take time before any effect may be manifest. Even allowing for such uncertainties, it is estimated in Europe that substantial proportions of the population are exposed to environmental factors that are a potential risk to health. While the most common outcomes are mild illnesses, some may have serious consequences. The priority remains to reduce exposure to such environmental hazards.

DEMOGRAPHY

Ageing in Europe is recognised as having implications for health. The demographic background is important in understanding the present and future health situation. Today Ireland has a relatively young population in European terms; however, the most striking result of population projections in the next thirty years is the increase in the number of persons aged sixty-five years and over. This represents an increase of almost 300,000 in those over sixty-five years, and the population aged eighty years and over will double over the projection period. The population is also projected to contain fewer young persons than there are at present. These demographic changes are likely to have a significant impact on both the need for and the nature of the services to be provided in future years.

TRENDS IN MORTALITY

Ireland, in comparison with most Western European countries, has experienced a reduction in mortality over the past fifty years. Recent trends indicate that mortality rates are continuing to decrease and there appears to be no reason to doubt that this decline should continue. The reasons for this decline are only partially understood. The general improvement in economic and social standards over the past fifty years has played an important part in reducing mortality. Effective health services, relating to prevention and care, have also contributed towards this better outcome. Preventive services have especially reduced mortality amongst infants and children, particularly in the area of infectious diseases. The differences in mortality from infectious diseases between 1947 and today are striking and marked reductions, including the elimination of several infectious diseases, have been achieved. The recent emergence of AIDS serves as a reminder that we cannot become complacent regarding infectious diseases. The trends in AIDS mortality are set to continue for a number of years; however, improved prevention and treatment programmes are likely to reduce the burden of this infectious disease in the longer term. The reduction of infectious disease mortality in infancy and childhood has been due largely to effective immunisation programmes. In many European countries, mortality during infancy and childhood is now so low that further reductions will be both very difficult and expensive to achieve. Congenital abnormalities are now the major causes of death and, even if all deaths during this period could be significantly reduced, this would result in negligible increases in overall life expectancy.

Improvements in life expectancy reflect the age specific mortality pattern as a whole. In the 1980s the major factor which increased life expectancy by 1.7 years in Europe was the reduction in mortality from cardiovascular diseases, particularly in older people. Reductions in mortality due to respiratory diseases and accidents also contributed to this increase in life expectancy. Despite Ireland's recent decline in cardiovascular and respiratory mortality, our rates are higher than the European Union average and there is therefore scope for improvement. Continued improvements in these areas will move Irish life expectancy towards the best in Europe. While it is difficult to predict trends in life expectancy, future improvements will primarily depend on mortality reductions in the middle-aged and elderly populations. Overall cancer mortality in Europe is rising and this will have a negative impact on life expectancy. It is hoped that this trend will be reversed by health promotion programmes and also by screening and early treatment which can reduce mortality from several types of cancer, including cancer of the breast and the cervix.

Improvements in screening techniques and extensive programmes for the early detection and treatment not only of cancer but of other chronic diseases such as hypertension and diabetes may also be expected to significantly reduce mortality and morbidity in the future. More effective healthcare can result from technological and treatment advances, both of which are likely to be expensive, and from delivering appropriate treatment to those likely to benefit from it. Advances in many areas have led to improved treatment and a slow but steady reduction in premature mortality from various conditions. It is expected that such progress will be maintained and that major advances may be made in some areas, such as gene therapy, which will yield significant benefits in the years to come.

In future years, further economic progress is likely; however, the rate of such progress is difficult to predict. Sustained economic progress has the effect of improving housing and nutrition status and living conditions generally, and increasing life expectancy. The size of these increases will depend on how equitably improvements in economic circumstances are distributed in the general population. Recent studies have pointed to economic segregation as an independent risk factor for health. Unemployment and social disadvantage are now recognised as a risk to health, exacerbating conditions such as cardiovascular disease, cancer and injuries. This is a major challenge facing many European countries. Economic progress is also linked to the health status of the population. Healthy children form the basis of the future of the country and a healthy adult population improves the productivity and welfare of the country in addition to reducing the costs of sick leave and premature retirement. Health and equitable economic development are closely linked, and the rate of health and social gain will be influenced by economic circumstances in future years.

We have seen significant progress in health status and new trends in healthcare in Ireland over the past fifty years. Despite these successes, there is scope for further improvement in future years. Today's priorities, namely to promote health and prevent the occurrence of disease, to improve people's environment and to improve health services, are similar to those of fifty years ago. There is a continuing need to improve health-related aspects of lifestyle, environmental conditions and healthcare in general. The recent *Health Strategy* reflects these concerns and points the way towards maximising health and social gain for the Irish population up to and beyond the year 2000.

CHAPTER 3

Promoting Health

Cecily Kelleher

INTRODUCTION

In the half century since the Department of Health was established in the Republic of Ireland, the field of social medicine and health education has changed out of all recognition. While the contribution of new technologies has facilitated huge changes in the delivery of health care to those already sick or with established disease, in a quieter way the scope for disease prevention, health promotion and health maintenance generally has been given new credibility by the vastly improved techniques for the study of health and disease status, coupled with the means for mass education about health. This paper proposes to explore some of these issues in an international and an Irish context and to examine the profound influences on health policy arising from this.

In 1990 the chair of health promotion was established in Galway with funding from the Department of Health. This was a highly innovative development, not just in Irish terms but internationally, since there are very few dedicated academic centres of health promotion and only a handful of academic professorships worldwide. Since then there has been a range of policy developments at national level, including the launch of the strategy document *Shaping a Healthier Future* and subsequently a specific health promotion document, *Making the Healthier Choice the Easier Choice*. There has been a number of government reports over the last decade from various expert committees which have focused, for instance, on the needs of specific groups such as women, travellers, older people, or those with disabilities. In each case the policy approach has been broad-ranging and often holistic, recognising the context in which people make health choices.

It is remarkable for physicians like me, trained in the seventies and taking up permanent posts in the nineties, to re-read the details of the controversies in the late 1940s and early 1950s about the entitlements of people to primary care and health education services, and the perceived dilemmas about individual freedom and moral responsibility advanced at the time (Barrington, 1987). Yet the issues of responsibility for personal health and well-being and personal control over health and lifestyle remain at the heart of modern health promotion and are basic tenets of the Ottawa Charter for Health Promotion (1986). On the one hand we are aware of the huge importance of personal living standards and lifestyle in determining health status and hence of the need in public policy terms to reach people early and constructively with public health messages. On the other hand there are those who consider the targeting of individuals about their lifestyle as victim blaming and who believe that the so-called Nanny State has overstepped its brief (Skrabanek and McCormack, 1989). This is perhaps most important now at a time when public policy is more clearly oriented than ever towards health promotion. Yet how valid is such criticism?

HEALTH GAIN IN THE LAST FIFTY YEARS

There is no doubt that in examining traditional health indicators such as morbidity and mortality we have made considerable progress in the last half century. Overall life expectancy has improved for both men and women and infant mortality has continued to decline, with figures for many of the indicators in the first year of life as good as those anywhere in the developed world, including neonatal and perinatal mortality (Central Statistics Office, personal communication). Considering we have had higher fertility rates than any of our European neighbours these are remarkable achievements. Undoubtedly however we export our problems as well. Our demographic picture as reflected in the population pyramid in the mid-1980s reflected the emigration patterns of the 1940s and 1950s, so we have a smaller older population than other countries, although in absolute terms that population is growing and will require greater support (Dept. of Labour Statistics, 1990). Our older people were economically better off than our neighbours and until recently had more family infrastructure for carer support (Kelleher, 1993). That may be set to change due to alterations in our family structure. Like all developed countries we will need to meet the challenge of a relatively older population profile in the future.

A closer look at our health statistics is more worrying, however. Life expectancy for older men has not improved since the 1920s (Fahey *et al*, 1993) and we have, relatively speaking, among the highest cardiovascular disease and cancer rates in the world for both men and women. There is reason to believe too that for a variety of genetic, cultural and environmental reasons Irish emigrants to Britain have poorer overall health status (Harding and Balarjan, 1996). Accordingly, in relative terms, much needs to be done to improve the health status of the Irish population as a whole and some sub-sections in particular if we are to have a standard of health comparable with our European neighbours, and indeed with the two great English-speaking economies of the world with a substantial ethnic Irish contribution, the US and Australia. The Irish lifestyle must be relevant. To take just one example, factors like alcohol behaviour are important, and full of paradoxes in that we have a high teetotaller population and quite respectable per capita consumption rates (Dept. of Health, 1996). However, in the recent UK study cited above, those Irish who do drink tend to drink more than other people. Here in Ireland in recent years we have seen changes in the social pattern of alcohol consumption, some with good consequences and some not so good. For instance there is more widespread acceptance of drink-driving legislation, an apparent decline of the round system and signs of more consumption of wine with meals (NNSC, 1993). On the other hand more people are drinking regularly and the key pattern of interest is the rise in serious alcohol-related illness in women, correlated with increased per capita consumption (Keogh and Walsh, 1996).

THE EMPHASIS ON IMPROVING INFRASTRUCTURE 1950-80

The history of the Irish health service is a fascinating one. Undoubtedly the reforms in primary care over a thirty-year period which facilitated public health nursing services, and the streamlining of GP services, helped to improve the health of the nation (Barrington, 1987). At the same time more fundamental factors such as food availability and improved nutrition also played their part, as can be seen in improved anthropometric indicators (NNSC, 1993). Adequate secondary and tertiary care services also emerged. In common with other developed countries we continued to develop our hospital services, and the emerging technologies in diagnostic and therapeutic fields helped to fuel these developments. We had peculiarly Irish factors at play in the development of our health services as well. As Barrington points out, the stock of buildings inherited from the post-famine period ensured a county hospital network which was stoutly maintained at local level for socio-economic as well as purely medical reasons (Barrington, 1987). The further drive towards infra-structure development in the fifties also meant a large stock of hospital beds and an inclination towards institutional rather than community care. The fact that our two-tiered health service tended to sponsor comprehensive coverage in the hospital rather than the community setting and that our health insurance scheme, unlike models in the United States, did not support health maintenance and primary care insurance also tended to protract our dependence on a hospital service structure (Commission on Health Services Funding, 1989).

The community care service has become highly sophisticated over the last twenty-five years but in practice has had little liaison with the general practice structure, making seamless care an impossibility. Approaches advocated in the UK in the late 1980s as in the Griffiths report would be impossible here (Murphy, 1990). In that system, the resource for care provision goes with the patient but since there is at present no co-ordinated hospital and community care structure that is impractical here. There are signs of change, however, particularly in initiatives to co-ordinate services for the elderly, who after all are proportionately the largest users of the health service and require multi-discipline and cross-sectoral support (Kelleher, 1993). In ascending order of priority, service provision for the already sick must precede preventive or screening services and health maintenance generally, and there has to be a culture of acceptance for primary care delivery. Sadly, we know very little about public attitudes to services in any systematic way, though if advertisement campaigns such as that initiated by the Office for Health Gain on appropriate utilisation of accident and emergency services are any indication, there is still a rooted support for hospital services as the main priority in the public mind. This is not so different in the UK, as a recent survey there also showed high priority for the mercifully rare but emotive conditions such as childhood leukaemia and rather less emphasis on preventive services (Bowling, 1996).

THE EMERGING SCIENCE OF EPIDEMIOLOGY

Perhaps no other factor has been more important in the shift towards health promotion and disease prevention than the development of epidemiology as a biomedical science since the end of the last world war. Epidemiology is the study of the determinants and distribution of disease in human populations. In quantitative terms, in modern developed countries the current plagues are of chronic diseases such as cardiovascular disease and cancers, followed by factors such as accidents. A hundred years ago in Europe the patterns of disease were similar to those seen now in the developing world, particularly the burden of infectious diseases (McKeown, 1976). While we became complacent about infectious disease in societies like ours, during the 1970s the emergence of the AIDS syndrome, patterns of resistant tuberculosis and now difficulties such as MRSA (methicillin resistant *staphylococcus aureus*) in institutional settings have reminded us of the precarious host-environment balance for all disease patterns. Epidemiology is concerned with time, space and person. As the epidemiologist Geoffrey Rose put it (Rose, 1985), why this person, of this disease, at this time? General characteristics of particular individuals or populations can predispose them to risk from particular conditions if the circumstances are right. Accordingly epidemiology is a science of probability, and public health advice is a way of alerting individuals to factors that may be modifiable and that they may wish therefore to modify to reduce risk. It is not like a clinical prescription for a treatment which we guarantee to work. Rather it is a method of support and advice.

What we have learnt from epidemiology about the causes of heart disease and all kinds of cancers is enormous. It has not yet told us everything but it has told us enough to ensure that coherent general guidelines can be put in place. Increasingly these principles have come to be applied in more clinical settings too, as for instance in the management of diabetes and established coronary heart disease and as a way of assessing best practice, so-called evidence-based medicine (Sackett *et al.*, 1996) So our debt to this science is considerable if sometimes underestimated. The success of good epidemiology is no outcome at all, and again as Geoffrey Rose indicated his main objective is to have no patient at all, grateful or otherwise. In Ireland epidemiology has been strong; the UCD/St Vincent's cardiology group was foremost in the world in the 1960s and 1970s in this field (Hickey *et al.*, 1975) and even today pioneers like Professor Ian Graham have continued to identify new and potentially important risk factors such as homocystenuria (Graham and Meleady, 1996). We also have had our contribution from those who warn us about the importance of proper and comprehensive evaluation of interventions like screening before their widespread application (Skrabanek and McCormack, 1989). Epidemiology is therefore a matter of enthusiasm, curiosity and innovation but also of caution and reason.

ACCEPTABILITY OF HEALTH PROMOTION AND DISEASE PREVENTION MESSAGE

In the last half century, but most particularly in the last twenty years, the health education and health promotion message has been widely disseminated and, I would contend, has been largely acceptable to most people most of the time. Popular interest in health, alternative and conventional medicine is an enormous media growth industry and indeed world-wide preoccupation with health, fitness and the leisure industry generally has been enormous. In a recent provocative article, Dr Ilona Kickbusch of the World Health Organisation documented the importance of the mass media industry generally in creating demand for information and entertainment and in promoting the growth of such discussion (Kickbusch, 1996). There have been corresponding trends which might be generalised to be most apparent for the better-off middle-class people in the developed world. Tobacco continues to be the largest single lifestyle problem in the developed world, with persistent rates of current smokers around a third of the population (Sixsmith, 1996). Yet in the 1960s a majority of men smoked and there was no real social class difference in that pattern (Phillips *et al.*, 1996). Nowadays that number has reduced by nearly a sixth among upper middle-class men, which is an extraordinary change. Though people find it hard to reduce fat intake there is considerable evidence of discretion being exercised in type of fat consumed, both in terms of specific commodities like butter and in high risk or motivated groups (NNSC, 1993: Thorogood *et al.*, 1990). The rates of personal leisure exercise among middle class women are higher than for their mothers and the rise in factors such as breastfeeding in women, particularly in the higher social classes, has been remarkable in most countries, although Ireland still has much lower rates (Becker and Kelleher, in prep.). Self-medication of aspirin for middle-aged men is now very common, the health food and alternative medicine industries are thriving and fear of environmental hazards in food can cripple an industry through consumer boycott, as seen in the recent BSE crisis. Accordingly it is erroneous to say that public health messages are not working. What we can say is that we often fail systematically to prove how they are working and have not always taken account of the other cultural determinants influencing such trends, some of which we welcome and some of which we do not. The role of public health education in providing proper information to facilitate informed choice is critically important. As with the parable of the half-empty or half-full glass, perhaps we should be studying more why health gains have been achieved than why they have not, as this may be a better formula for success.

EMERGING DILEMMAS WORLD-WIDE

To a large degree Irish public health policy has been innovative and evidence-based for some years. *Health the Wider Dimensions*, a policy document from the mid-eighties, was novel in recognising the need for rational, need-driven services and the recognition that the determinants of health are broadly based. The strategy document produced nearly a decade later was praised for retaining that comprehensive spirit, and unlike *The Health of the Nation* in the UK for not placing the onus mainly on the health care delivery sector to promote individual health gain. However, there is always a danger of establishing rational strategic plans that cannot deliver in practice. Some of the problems that arise include resistance to change and competition for scarce resources by existing service providers, lack of preparedness on the part of the general public for new thinking, particularly where shortcomings in existing services are highlighted, and factors other than health need that dictate the existing infrastructure.

Finally, and most critically, is lack of resources. It is a complex business to decide what and how much should be spent on health services. We fare respectably by international standards in the amount we spend overall on our health service, but by any standards based on need, our budget on preventive services is limited. The Kilkenny Health Project was established in 1985 and reflected a climate of spontaneous change in lifestyle and raised awareness about risk factors for coronary heart disease (Shelley *et al.*, 1995). Indeed in political terms resources could not have been so deployed in a publicly funded health service if there were not public goodwill towards its objectives. That project achieved its aims. However, spontaneous health gain, probably for similar reasons, also took place in the reference county. The real test of an intervention project is how well it fares with targeted subgroups most likely to avail of a service and how in the long-term those changes are sustained. The budget for the Kilkenny project was modest, however, and world-wide, even in the last half dozen years, we are seeing considerably more sophisticated understanding of what is likely to influence behaviour change in a mass setting or in more focused settings, such as schools, workplaces or small communities.

Increasingly what has been disturbing about health status are the major inequalities emerging between countries and within countries according to socio-demographic patterns, as highlighted recently in the UK (Smith, 1997). It is possible to change behaviour, but this extends to health maintenance practice generally and not just personal lifestyle. Health is a matter of politics as much as personal practice. If one has access to education, is personally content and secure in one's work and family, has the kind of personality that predisposes to believing in personal control over life circumstances and likely success in changing those circumstances, if one trusts and understands the motivation and content of the message, then such an individual will be likely to take care of his or her health by changing lifestyle and asserting rights to a proactive health care service. If this is not generally true of the circumstances then he or she will not. To understand all these factors we need the skills and methodologies of the social scientists, anthropologists, sociologists, psychologists and economists. Quantitative methods can tell us how many people need help, qualitative methods will tell us whether they will successfully avail of that help. The recognition that what might appear intuitively obvious may also be sophisticated to prove and deliver is the modern challenge of health care delivery. Clearly, health inequalities tell us that for some reason we are failing as a society. Complex analysis tells us simply that complex problems are not solved by single strategies and over-simplification.

Finally there is an ethical dimension to health promotion and health service delivery generally. We must value good health as a society and agree the price to be paid for it before we can plan for and implement services. For the extreme civil libertarian, it is not enough to establish that a health behaviour is harmful if that person asserts the right to such a choice. For the religious person, the common good may not be put before the dignity of the individual person. For the social change reformer, the notion may also be unacceptable that society sustains inequalities that discriminate against the most needy because those individuals apparently do not perceive their own need. These are fine moral questions, but over the last half century we have in effect moved to a more populist position that assumes services primarily based on need and we expect that principle to apply generally, irrespective of means. Health economics has taught us, however, that we cannot endlessly or aimlessly provide services just because we can do so; we have to direct services where they are best utilised, a matter of some discussion and concern in modern Ireland.

THE IRISH SITUATION

The more recent history of health education in Ireland dates to the mid-seventies when a national Health Education Bureau (HEB) was established (Hensey, 1988). This achieved a relatively high media profile in its early years and was responsible for developing links between Ireland and other countries in this field, for a number of high profile conferences and research collaborations and for the sponsoring of various, particularly media-based, campaigns. The Bureau, however, had few formal links with the executive agencies and in effect most of the health boards developed their own health education programmes, particularly with the schools. The two major national voluntary organisations, the Irish Cancer Society and the Irish Heart Foundation, also developed various programmes which continued to expand, particularly in relation to lifestyle education and smoking cessation. Then in 1986 a working party set up through the HEB to examine the issue of health education and health promotion produced a report entitled *Promoting Health*

Through Public Policy (HEB, 1987), which stressed the need for concerted co-ordinated action across a range of sectors if meaningful changes in risk factor profiles for the major avoidable diseases were to be achieved. The report set the scene for significant change. The HEB was disbanded and within the Department of Health itself a new unit was established. This health promotion unit (HPU) in effect took over much of the education and information dissemination role of its predecessor the HEB, but also functioned as an executive as well as a policy-making unit and was intended to establish closer practical links with the health boards. A new cabinet subcommittee for health promotion was formed comprising relevant ministries influencing health status, though in fact this group never met in plenary. Some significant decisions were taken under its auspices, including negotiation on AIDS education materials intended for second-level schools, and discussions on a voluntary smoking ban in the workplace. A national Advisory Council on Health Promotion was established and over the next six years three advisory councils were convened, chaired successively by two presidents of the Royal College of Physicians, Professor Ivo Drury and Dr Ciaran Barry, and finally by Frances Fitzgerald, later a member of Dail Éireann. The council worked on a range of policy documents and reports in subcommittee format. Its work was important behind the scenes but it achieved little profile or publicity in itself. Two of the subcommittees subsequently generated a *National Alcohol Policy* (Dept. of Health, 1996A) and *Recommendations for a National Food Policy for Ireland* (Nutrition Advisory Group, 1995). With the production of *Shaping a Healthier Future* specific health promotion targets were formulated and a new cross-sectoral advisory group was formulated to replace the old council, now chaired by the responsible Junior Minister for Health, Brian O'Shea TD.

At health board level throughout the period, activity continued. This account is not intended to be exhaustive, but I mention here some examples of work with which I am familiar. The North Western Health Board evaluated its extensive lifeskills schools programme after a decade's work (Nic Gabhainn and Kelleher, 1995), and the Mid-Western Health Board continued to expand its education programme for schools, as did the Southern Health Board. The Western Health Board built up a successful community facilitation network and the South Eastern Health Board built on the experience of the Kilkenny Health Project. There was considerable health promotion activity in various areas and divisions in the Eastern Health Board, notably in collaboration with the local authorities in the WHO Healthy Cities Project. All the health boards now have some kind of explicit health promotion policy.

The final most significant development during 1994 to 1996 was the appointment at senior managerial level of health promotion officers in virtually all the boards, and the appointment of new directors of public health with responsibility for population surveillance and planning for appropriate health care delivery.

DRAWBACKS TO PROGRESS

The national strategy of health advocates an outcome-based system under the general headings of health and social gain. It follows that within each disciplinary area and for each service in the health sector, specific targets need to be formulated, to be achieved within a set time scale and evaluated appropriately. The strategy document reflects this across a range of services and there are eight specific targets in the health promotion area in relation to modifiable risk factors. In order to measure such achievement, however, needs assessment has to be undertaken and measures of health status agreed. This is one of the traditional deficiencies now being rectified at national and health board level. Once we have agreed a common dataset and, crucially, begun to collect lifestyle and attitudinal data systematically, we should be in a strong position to promote and achieve evidence-based health services. While we need to be outcome-driven the optimum process for effective and efficient delivery also has to be evaluated. Such rigour need not generate a bureaucratic albatross for health care providers if it is well integrated and automatic in planning a service.

At the time the Department of Health Promotion was set up in 1990 at University College Galway (UCG), there was virtually no pertinent research material on these issues available in the country. The Kilkenny Health Project was part of the international MONICA (Multinational MONItoring of trends and determinants in CArdiovascular disease) surveillance system but we had no national morbidity data set. Since then in UCG we have undertaken a range of relevant work. From the beginning we have taken a broad definition of health promotion and have applied its principles in a range of activities and settings. In 1992 with Department of Health support we established a national nutrition surveillance centre which collated and co-ordinated information on all aspects of the food chain and diet-related health impact (NNSC, 1993). This work is now being expanded at UCG to include broader lifestyle and behavioural surveillance. Ireland is one of the foremost countries in Europe in relation to diet and nutrition research with a strong profile in several of the universities.

In addition we have conducted a number of needs assessment projects, examining attitudes to a variety of issues, for example perceived risk of cardiovascular disease (Nic Gabhainn and Kelleher, 1996), attitudes of women to mammography services (Sixsmith, 1995) and attitudes of older people to their health and well-being (Murphy, in prep.). We have also conducted a number of health services research projects, on health needs of travellers (Dept. of Health, 1996b), of carers (O'Donovan *et al.,* 1997), of general practice service provision. Finally we have an active settings intervention and evaluation programme, of the workplace (Hope and Kelleher, 1995), general practice and schools (Nic Gabhainn and Kelleher, 1995).

UCG is by no means the only research centre conducting relevant work. Again it is not possible to be exhaustive but work conducted by the Economic and Social Research Institute (ESRI), the Marino Institute and others for the Health Promotion Unit has been of relevance to the schools projects particularly. This active research and evaluation programme of health promotion was needed if health policy in this area is to be based properly on appropriate evidence. We have also had in UCG an active role in training and education of health and education sector professional involved in health education and programmes, at adult and continuing education level, at undergraduate, postgraduate and post-professional level (Dineen and Kelleher, 1995). The establishment of an independent academic chair of health promotion was hence novel and innovative on the part of the Department of Health and in keeping with its stated policy objectives in this area, over the last decade in particular.

PROJECTIONS FOR THE NEW MILLENNIUM

So, where to from here for the Irish health services, and for the Department of Health in particular? In 1947 the establishment of a specific department and ministry with responsibility for health represented recognition for the success in health care delivery and the emerging biotechnical sciences. There are drawbacks to achieving health and well-being for the nation as a whole if the heath service is primarily a sickness service and if there is no input on health matters in public policy generally. Good health is crucially dependent on conducive public policy across the socio-cultural spectrum. However, it would be absurd not to recognise the need for a well-structured coherent health care delivery service. In Ireland we have kept a broader sense of the relationship between social, physical and mental aspects to health and well-being than other countries, both at a strategic level in our most recent policy documents and at an operational level in the links at community care level with environmental and social welfare services. We are rare in Europe in emphasising the cross-sectoral influences on health and in keeping those principles enshrined in our national mission statement (Dept. of Health, 1994). The newest changes proposed for the health services involve further devolution regionally and a strengthened objective-driven service management. It is too early to say what the implications are of these changes and it would be naive not to recognise the complexity involved in realising some of the aspirations above, but at least we have a framework to contend with and debate.

An ideal society is one where health inequalities are minimised, where treatment services are mainly deployed to deal with ageing and death and where high technology is focused on the diseases that are truly not preventable. To strive to achieve this is part of the challenge of being human. There is no excuse for not starting because we think we cannot finish. Undoubtedly health promotion is here to stay for two reasons, in my view. Firstly, knowledge about the potential to prevent ill health is at least as good as that about the potential to treat, and this is the message for the education of all health professionals in the next century. Secondly, people in society generally are better informed than ever before about their rights and responsibilities in relation to their health.

Enormous global challenges face all of us in relation to the vast world population and we should realise that more people die now on this earth every day from famine, pestilence and war than at any time in human history. On the other hand if we just confine our horizons to Ireland, from Donegal to Cork, from Wexford to Ballina, then the children being born now should expect at the very least to see an end to some of the avoidable disease patterns afflicting their grandparents. We have the means, the motive and the opportunity; what we need is the determination to succeed.

CHAPTER 4

The Role of General Practice in a Developing Health Service

Michael Boland

EVOLUTION OF IRISH GENERAL PRACTICE

General practice occupies a key position in the Irish health care system. For most patients their general practitioner (GP) is their 'point of first contact' with the system. Most illness is diagnosed and most prescribing occurs in general practice. Fitness for work, fitness to drive, legal competence and many of the other entitlements of illness are certified by the GP. GPs are a major source of individual health education and personal behaviour and lifestyle advice. Most significantly in terms of cost, patient access to secondary and tertiary care services is largely through referral by a GP.

Irish general practice has its origins in the poor law system established in the middle of last century to provide relief to the poor and destitute. The cost of the services was to be derived from local rates. The country was divided into 'Unions' or small districts and their services were confined at first to 'workhouses', built and operated harshly with the specific intention of discouraging anyone from using them unless driven by dire need.

Later the rules were relaxed so that 'outdoor' relief was provided outside the confines of the workhouse. This led to the appointment of district medical officers (DMOs) who assumed responsibility for all eligible patients in the district. Initially this GP service was geographically based, patients had no choice of doctor, and the intention was to discourage use. Payment of the doctors by salary provided no incentive to increase their workload. Patients attended often rudimentary local 'dispensaries' for consultation and basic treatment. House calls were made to those unable to attend. Only in the 1950s were patient lists introduced.

Most DMOs complemented their stipends by developing a private practice in the locality. It was typically quite distinct from the dispensary service; private patients were seen in another location (often the doctor's home), were given more time, and paid the doctor in cash at each visit. Often they had a choice of doctor.

It was this two-tiered system and the lack of choice for the dispensary patients which prompted the introduction of the 'fee per item of service' contract with GPs in 1972.

Meanwhile health administration in Ireland had altered radically. Under the Health Services (Financial Provisions) Act 1947, rates ceased to be the major source of funding, and the state undertook to raise its share of health service costs from 16% to 50%. The Voluntary Health Insurance Board (VHI) was set up in 1957. Debate in the 1960s culminated in the Health Act of 1970. The 1966 White Paper proposed the transfer of administration from the local authorities to regional boards whose membership would 'represent a partnership between local government, central government, and the vocational organisations.'

The justification for change was that an increasing proportion of funds were by now derived from the centre. The growing complexity of techniques and equipment required economies of scale. Over 50% of all inpatients in acute hospitals in 1966 were treated in large teaching and regional hospitals. Community and GP services might have remained with local authorities but for the importance of maintaining unitary control. Unfortunately GP services remained effectively outside the new health board system at that time, setting the stage for a quite separate development of community-based public health, nursing and social services. This lack of a unified community health service persists today, although the development in the last five years of GP units in the health boards and the employment of GPs as unit advisors have been very positive moves towards unity.

From 1972 GP services have been funded in an unusual way. Thirty-six percent of the population are entitled to all services, including prescriptions, free of charge. Their eligibility is determined mostly by means testing, although many patients with chronic illness and most of the elderly are included. The remainder of the population pay the GP on a fee per item of service basis. This creates a 'poverty trap', discouraging those whose incomes narrowly exceed the eligibility limit from attending for screening and long-term care. It also creates a perverse incentive for the 65% of the population who must pay the GP because secondary care in hospitals is either free or less expensive for the user.

FEE FOR SERVICE SYSTEM

The 'fee per item of service' system was administered nationally by the General Medical Services (Payments) Board (GMS). Eligible patients were free to choose a doctor from a panel of participating doctors in their locality. Increasingly GPs developed single surgery premises so that all patients, whether public or private, were seen at one location without distinction. GPs were paid a fee for each item of service they provided (surgery visit, home visit, out of hours service, etc.). This payment system and competition for patients ensured that patient satisfaction with the system was high and the level of patient complaint extremely low. Therefore in terms of the problems that it sought to address the 1972 GMS contract was a success.

However, the system was more costly to operate than had been anticipated and these costs rose steadily over the years until 1989, when the system changed. The increases were attributable to a rise in the number of eligible patients and a rise in the average number of consultations per patient per year. Interestingly the number of GPs holding contracts also increased to the extent that the average earnings per doctor (adjusted for inflation) remained constant for the duration of the contract.

From the management point of view, however, the constant rise in clinical activity was unsustainable. More consultations meant more prescriptions and the cost of prescribing accounted for more than two-thirds of the annual GMS budget. Worst of all it proved impossible to predict with any precision by how much the budget would grow in future years.

From the professional point of view also the fee-per-item of service contract had some disadvantages. There were no proper and separate provisions for practice expenses, pension and sick leave allowances, and capital investment in premises and equipment. The contract was a global payment intended to include everything. In reality for many GPs current costs absorbed all available funds.

THE CURRENT PAYMENT SYSTEM

For these reasons a new GMS contract was agreed with the profession in 1989 based on a capitation system of payment. For each patient the doctor received an annual fee, adjusted for the age and location of the patient. Allowances covering the cost of pensions, sick leave, holiday locums, etc. were also paid according to list size. A limited number of special services attracted a fee per item of service. Together these accounted for less than 5% of total income. Later other allowances were added to encourage the employment of practice nurses and secretaries. Many of the problems associated with the previous contract were thus addressed.

The main disadvantage of the current GMS contract is that it lacks performance-related incentives. Unfortunately no systematic evaluation is available to indicate whether the contract changes resulted in a reduction in doctors' clinical activity (fewer house calls, fewer out of hours calls, less repeat visiting by those with chronic illness, or more referral).

The area of prescribing is the only area of activity for which comprehensive reliable data do exist. Such was the continuing rise in both the volume and cost of prescribed drugs that a further initiative was required to bring it under control, and the GPs and the Department of Health agreed to the introduction of a drug budgeting scheme for all GMS doctors. Each GP was given a personal prescribing target based on their current level of prescribing and the projected cost for the coming year. Those who reached their targets were entitled to claim a 'drug refund' equivalent to 50% of the notional savings made for use in improving the practice premises or equipment, or in pursuing approved professional development. The remaining 50% of savings were made available at national or health board level for the development of general practice.

The drug budgeting scheme has been amongst the most successful schemes in Europe in achieving its targets. This has been attributed to the intensive promotion campaign undertaken annually by the Irish Medical Organisation. While no published impact study is available to evaluate the effect on quality of care, the overall impression is that there has been no serious adverse effect.

Patients not entitled to GMS services should be entitled to cover their costs using private medical insurance. Two companies (VHI and BUPA) operate in Ireland and do offer subscribers a GP benefit package. However the initial co-payment is set at a level which requires the subscriber to attend the GP more than twenty times a year before any benefit applies. This ensures that less than 3% of the population can ever claim.

IRISH COLLEGE OF GENERAL PRACTITIONERS

The foundation of the Irish College of General Practitioners in 1984 provided for the first time a co-ordinated approach to the development of general practice as an unique discipline in medicine. The aims of the college were to maintain the highest possible standards of care for patients through improved training, education and research. GPs strongly supported the development and more than 95% of established GPs became foundation members. Within three years a membership examination was established and within eight years a comprehensive set of training programmes was in place. The existing small group CME network was incorporated and extended to all parts of the country. National scientific meetings, a regular college journal, and a wide range of standing committees, task groups, regional research advisors and project fellowships complete a picture of intense academic activity.

The establishment in 1997 of a Postgraduate Resource Centre to co-ordinate and further develop these activities represents a new and exciting chapter in the life of the college. It has been made possible by financial support from the Department of Health through the GMS. As such it represents an historic partnership between government and profession in the development of general practice.

A recent ICGP survey of Irish General Practice (1996) will prove to be among its most significant achievements. It has identified 2200 GPs in full-time or substantial part-time practice. For a total population of 3.6 million this indicates an average list size of 1,635 patients per doctor. At a consultation rate of 4.5 visits per patient per annum, the average GP has twenty-eight 'face to face' consultations per day. At the rate of five consultations per hour s/he spends six hours consulting per day. The total number of GP consultations in Ireland annually is thus estimated to be 16.2 million.

GENERAL PRACTICE AND THE CHALLENGES FOR HEALTH CARE

Containing cost has become the overwhelming challenge for health care systems. Annual spending on health care as estimated by the World Bank in 1990 shows the USA at one extreme with US$2763 per capita. It seems that there is no limit to the amount which can be spent on health. Contrast this with the countries of sub-Saharan Africa where annual spending is less than US$10 per capita. Europe lies somewhere in between, with the specialist-dominated countries of Scandinavia, France and Germany heading the list. The British 'primary care led' national health service is notably cost-effective. That year it cost 6.0% of UK GNP in contrast to 12.2% of GNP spent by the United States. Ireland at that time spent a relatively modest US$876, although this represented 8.6% of GNP.

More recently in Ireland the rising cost of health care has been a cause for concern. Over the last five years, while the general price index rose by only 15% (3% per annum), current spending on health rose by 65% and capital spending by 143% – a trend which one notable Irish economist described as 'unsustainable'.

Doctors cannot be immune to this challenge. It is no longer possible for them to adopt the high moral ground and say that patient need must always come before cost. Need is relative and satisfying the needs of one individual may only be possible by sacrificing the needs of another. Health service managers are entitled to expect doctors to achieve best value for money. At a minimum doctors should assist managers by clarifying the spending choices.

In Ireland access to specialist services is largely through referral by a general practitioner. Nevertheless a substantial proportion of admissions to hospital (30%) are arranged through their accident and emergency departments and only a third of these originate with a GP. It is an increasing source of frustration to GPs that these departments are used by the hospitals for pre-admission screening of referrals by relatively inexperienced young doctors.

In circumstances in which demand exceeds supply, rationing is required. This may be achieved by financial disincentives and waiting lists. These are blunt instruments which can cause great hardship to individual patients. More humane options include criteria based on need (capacity to benefit) and/or urgency, and more devolution of clinical responsibility to general practice.

The increasing level of activity in acute hospitals is the main source of rising cost. Medical practice is changing and paradoxically in some respects the hospital is 'shrinking'. Patient stay is getting shorter, day care is growing and more specialists are going to work in the community. In 1995 more than 160,000 day cases were handled in Irish hospitals. Yet as these changes occur, hospital workload is increasing.

For example a recent report (*British Medical Journal* Editorial April '96) confirmed that emergency admissions in Scotland between 1981 and 1994 rose by 45%. The author commented, 'with the exception of childhood asthma and self poisoning there is little evidence of any genuine rise in disease incidence'.

In Ireland total hospital outpatient attendances rose by 20% between 1982 and 1992 to reach 1.8 million per annum. The proportion of 'new' outpatient attendances has remained more or less constant at 20%. This suggests a proportionate and sustained increase in the number of patients being newly referred by their GPs.

Specialist practice is increasingly procedure-driven. In many countries specialists are regarded more highly and rewarded more generously for the five minutes they spend passing a fibreoptic scope than for the forty-five minutes they spend conducting a thorough history and examination. It seems to be more 'efficient' to investigate and manage patients in 'cohorts' than to care for them as individuals. There is a danger that this reduces the role of the doctor to that of a technician and professional identity is correspondingly diminished. The immediate challenge for GPs is not merely to counterbalance this form of medicine but to resist the inevitable pressure to copy it.

The wider challenge for general practice is to reverse recent trends and reduce the number of patients referred to acute hospitals for investigation and treatment. Any attempt to depart from the principle that access to specialist services should be through the GP must be strenuously resisted. A survey of Western Europe in 1992 revealed that GPs have this 'gatekeeper' role in only two-thirds of the countries included. Direct access to specialists is costly because it leads to unnecessary, inappropriate and premature interventions. It is also undesirable because it fragments care and may make patients unduly dependent and even neurotic about their health. However, even in countries where access to specialist services is through the GP, the 'medicalisation' of the population is proceeding apace. General practice must take some responsibility for this.

THE SPECTRUM OF HEALTH & HEALTH CARE

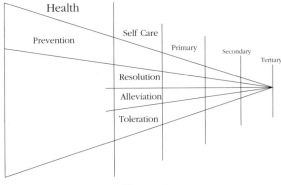

Figure 1

The state of the population's health and their position within the health care system may be regarded as a spectrum extending from full health at one end to tertiary care at the other (see Figure 1). Between these extremes are the bands of self care, primary care, and secondary care. Moving from 'health' on the left across the spectrum to 'tertiary care' on the right in each successive band, the proportion of the population falls steeply and both the cost and the degree of patient dependency rises.

In 1961 Kerr White, the great American pioneer of ambulatory care, published research on patient-reported illness. During a period of one month 1000 adults recorded their illness episodes and their contact with health services. Seven hundred and fifty reported one or more illnesses or injuries of whom one-third (250) consulted a doctor. Only nine were admitted to hospital and only one was referred to a tertiary centre.

A central objective of health care must be to move people always in the direction of health and to avoid drawing them into the system, particularly to levels of unnecessary specialisation. GPs have a pivotal role in such a system because they largely define two crucial boundaries – the boundary with specialist care and the boundary with self care.

THE BOUNDARY WITH SECONDARY CARE

There are approximately eight times as many GP consultations as there are outpatient attendances. An average GP will manage 96% of his/her consultations so that fewer than 4% of consultations result in a referral to a specialist. It is clear that even a marginal variation in referral behaviour – for example from 96% to 95% – would result in a 25% increase in the number of patients reaching hospital. The challenge for the hospital specialist must be to question in every case whether care could not be provided as safely and efficiently in general practice.

Equally the GP must question the real necessity for each referral. From an average GP list of 1650 patients in a single year 188 'new' patients are referred to a hospital outpatient clinic and there are 638 'old' OPD attendances. 237 patients from the practice are discharged from hospital and 85 are treated as 'day cases'. In addition practice patients account for 511 A&E Department attendances.

The most important prerequisite for efficient high quality referral is good communication between the specialist and GP, based on mutual respect. Regular contact allows agreement on the content of pre-referral work-up, agreed urgency criteria, and agreed discharge criteria. GPs should remain involved after referral, at least when strategic decisions regarding the patient's future are being taken, and there should be a common approach to 'carers'.

Another priority for GPs and specialists together must be to examine the potential for new forms of shared care, particularly for patients suffering from chronic illness. Long-term outpatient hospital clinics where more than 90% of the attendances are 'old' would be the most useful place to start. These include endocrine, haematology, and renal clinics. Specialists in these disciplines will need to be reassured that standards will be maintained after care has been shared. This can be achieved by clear protocols, combined care record cards and good communication.

Effective electronic links facilitating rapid and effortless transfer of clinical data between practices and hospitals will make it much easier to monitor shared care. Telemedicine may allow patients and GPs the benefit of a specialist opinion from the comfort of the local surgery. So-called 'near patient testing' can become more reliable if test findings are remotely reviewed by a specialist in difficult or doubtful cases.

THE BOUNDARY WITH SELF CARE

A central challenge for GPs must be to define the meaning of 'unmet need'. Patient needs are likely to become the measure by which all medical care will be judged. In reality, for every five patients seen in general practice, twenty-five more with symptoms causing them concern decided not to consult. One hundred more have symptoms which do not concern them.

All common conditions like anxiety/depression, arthritis, upper respiratory infections, and dyspepsia follow this pattern of the 'illness iceberg'. Were we to attempt to meet the needs of all these patients our systems would collapse. The challenge is to empower them to care for themselves and to educate them in the appropriate use of our services so that those who consult are the ones most likely to benefit. The same critical approach applied to the necessity for referral must be applied to patients attending their GPs. If GPs encourage more and more people to consult, more will also reach specialist care.

More than 90% of patient consultations with their GP are dealt with entirely by the doctor without referral for either diagnostic investigation or a specialist opinion. About 70% of the population will attend a GP at least once in any year and in five years more than 95% will do so. Irish patients consult their GPs on average four to five times per year. Ideally, patients should only consult their doctors when it is both appropriate and timely to do so. The extent to which they do this depends on their knowledge of the significance of symptoms and signs, and their understanding of the natural history of disease. Whilst this varies widely the overall impression is one of relative ignorance even amongst those well educated in all other aspects of living. Medical science should form a larger part of the general primary and secondary school curriculum.

News and current affairs media also have a heavy responsibility to inform the public. In particular when reporting sensational medical events or novel treatments their capacity to raise false hope or undue anxiety should caution them to apply the highest journalistic standards of scientific veracity to such reports.

In Ireland 80% of consultations result in a prescription. Some of these courses are never filled, consumed or completed. Many patients attend for reassurance. Yet although the real reason for consulting is fear of cancer, heart disease, or serious infection, what is presented to the doctor is a symptom (pain, tiredness etc.). This often leads the doctor to respond with reassurance and a prescription, when reassurance alone would have sufficed. To prevent this unnecessary prescribing both doctors and patients must come to accept that the presentation of concern alone and its treatment by reassurance alone is a legitimate part of healthcare.

Some patients on long-term medication (for example the contraceptive pill) and some who present with minor self-limiting illness could avoid attending the doctor entirely if some drugs were licensed for sale 'over the counter' (OTC). With better patient education there is considerable scope for more OTC drugs without any significant risk.

Once a patient presents to a doctor the presumption is that there is disease present until proven otherwise. In general practice the burden of proof depends on the gravity of the presumed disease and its probability in the context of positive and negative clinical findings. Whilst in general practice the probability of serious disease is fortunately low, the degree of uncertainty when relying on history and clinical examination alone is relatively high.

In the past the individual doctor decided the level of risk to the patient and the degree of uncertainty which s/he considered acceptable. As a matter of professional responsibility GPs kept this process of judgement and its accompanying doubts to themselves. Patients were offered clear definite advice and solid reassurance. Now many doctors prefer to involve the patient in the process of reaching a decision, sharing the responsibility but also the uncertainty. Some patients may find this approach less reassuring and demand more sophisticated testing and more referrals to specialists. However, the general tendency to less paternalism and the specific fear of litigation will ensure the trend continues, with the serious consequences of medicalisation and increased health care costs.

THE CONTENT AND VALUES OF GENERAL PRACTICE

We must remember our fundamental values as doctors as new developments seek to redefine them. We believe in the values of relevance, equity, quality, cost effectiveness, rationality and humanity. But privatisation may challenge equity; and cost effectiveness and quality may often conflict. Humane medicine may be forgotten in the enthusiasm for new technologies; and the rational basis of the increasingly bizarre methods of alternative practitioners may not be challenged because we do not wish to appear too superior. In all these debates relevance to patients should be our guiding light.

Stott and Davis (1979) described four areas in the exceptional potential in each primary care consultation: management of presenting problems, management of continuing problems, modification of help-seeking behaviour, opportunistic health promotion. The last two areas are often sacrificed to the pressing needs of the others. This may be as it should be. However GPs need to decide what strategies should be adopted to address the important issues of health education and behavioural advice.

The publication of a draft Charter of General Practice by the European office of WHO, setting out its most important characteristics, meets some of these challenges. The Charter underlines the fact that as GPs we are defined by the patients we look after. They are a population of named individuals and they constitute the 'content' of our expertise just as the diseases of children define a paediatrician or the diseases of the gut define a gastro-enterologist. It is important that every Irish citizen should be able to name his/her family doctor and every GP should have a full list of the patients for whom s/he is responsible. Loosely arranged private practice without formal patient registration makes that goal for the moment unattainable.

The absence of a list system in Ireland also has serious consequences for planning and policy making. We will never be in a position to judge the level of clinical activity of a GP (numbers of consultations, prescriptions or referrals) until we know the number of patients served by his/her practice. Without this 'foundation block' it is also impossible to construct a meaningful information system for the rest of the health service. A computerised information system capable of providing anonymous data in a standardised form is a national priority.

It has been written that GPs grow in expertise by seeing a series of illnesses in the same individual; other specialists grow in expertise by seeing the same diseases in a series of individuals. This makes general practice not just another speciality but a separate dimension of medical care. But how well do we know our patients, and can we organise and record that knowledge to enhance its value? If we are to understand our patients in context we must ask ourselves what we know of the patient's health beliefs, functional capacity, significant relationships, household, social supports, financial situation, and dependency. If we are to marshal community support on behalf of our patients we must ask ourselves what social networks we have.

The Charter stresses that general practice is 'general' in as much as it includes all sorts of problems and all sorts of people. It is 'personal' because it is based on a personal relationship and 'primary' because it is first contact care. It is 'comprehensive' because it combines the tasks of diagnosing, curing, caring, preventing, and educating the patient. It must be 'accessible' – available for use when needed, and affordable. It is 'continuing' both during and between episodes. It is 'high context' in the sense that care is modified by the patient's family, work, community etc. It has a 'co-ordinating' function – advising on, referring to, and monitoring specialist, hospital, and community services. It provides 'advocacy' by representing the patient's needs to others. It is 'collaborating' (working with other team members) and 'confidential' . It must be 'enabling', that is encouraging patients to be 'care free' and independent. It is 'certifying', officially confirming the patient' s status. Finally it is 'local' – defined by its geographical location.

To these core functions of general practice must be added competence. Southgate has identified two major components of competence: 'the consistent ability to select and perform tasks employing intellectual, psychomotor, and interpersonal skills' and 'the consistent demonstration of appropriate moral and personality attributes'. She further defines it as being '...in part the ability, in part the will to select and perform consistently, relevant clinical tasks in the context of the social environment in order to resolve health problems of individuals and groups in an efficient, effective, economic and humane manner'.

Quality professional performance requires values which motivate the competent doctor to perform optimally. As Marshall Marinker has written, 'General Practice is not only a biotechnical enterprise and a managerial challenge; it is also a moral endeavour' and, in a similar vein, McIntyre and Popper declare: '. . . efforts to improve performance must come from a desire for self-improvement, a desire based on an essentially ethical insight.'

GPs should welcome the inevitable progress towards recertification of doctors and reaccreditation of practices. We should insist however that the assessment of performance reflects the complexity of our professional task and is not based on trivial accumulation of credits and/or misleading indicators. Medical care may have many intended outcomes. These include problem resolution, symptom relief, and improved functional status. They also include preventing premature death, the effects of disease and disability, and the fear of illness. Less obviously perhaps patient satisfaction, doctor satisfaction, and enabling patients to achieve their potential are also important. Systems of quality assessment should reflect this wider picture.

THE EDUCATIONAL RESPONSE

It is now widely accepted that undergraduate or 'basic' medical education is no longer intended to produce a doctor capable of practice without further training. Instead the aim now is to produce a student who is broadly educated in medicine and ready for postgraduate training. The student should be capable of making an informed career choice and should still be strongly motivated for a life of service to patients. Ability to solve problems, to communicate effectively and to approach the patient with the appropriate ethical and moral attributes should be well established. Other key outcomes would be students who can self-direct their own lifelong learning, know how to use scientific method, and can critically appraise innovations in medical management as they emerge. Flexibility and effective team-working complete the picture of the well-educated medical student ready for postgraduate training.

Much progress has been made in Ireland in the last ten years in basic medical education in acknowledging the contribution which general practice can make. General Practice has been formally recognised as a specialist discipline by the Medical Council, and Chairs of General Practice have been established in all medical schools.

The stage is now set for a radical reform of the undergraduate curriculum in Ireland, such as is occurring in many of the world's great medical schools. GPs should support the Medical Council in this process. It is clear that effective basic medical education can only be achieved if community-based clinical teaching is developed. This requires the use of practice-linked programmes in the future but can only be realistic if properly funded. In practical terms this means that the same special funding increments provided to hospitals engaged in teaching in the past must now be made available to teaching practices. These increments were used to provide higher levels of staffing (and thus more time for senior staff to teach) and physical facilities to accommodate students. The student experience in such teaching practices must be active and structured and not mere passive observation of service professionals at work.

At the postgraduate level there are three phases in the education of a family doctor. Specific training of three years' duration at least is now accepted in Europe and the challenge will be to continually review each element of those years for relevance to subsequent practice. Methods of assessing the progress of registrars throughout the programme are also the subject of much debate. There is now a consensus amongst programme directors that the period of training needs to be extended to four years. This view is soundly based on more than five years' pilot study experience in the Sligo programme, which has been positive.

Following the training period it takes most doctors another five years to become fully acquainted with a community practice and establish a personal relationship with the patients named on his/her list. Continuity and personal care are not possible until this phase is complete. It may also be a time for the new GP to undertake special interests in research, quality assurance, and teaching.

In Ireland the years immediately following training are particularly difficult for newly-qualified GPs who must find employment wherever they can while awaiting a suitable practice vacancy. This is highly undesirable from every point of view and needs to be urgently addressed.

The final phase of education is continuing medical education (CME). In Ireland the scope of CME has been enlarged from its base in traditional lecture programmes to include active participation in small group learning by more than 70% of all GPs. These learning groups are supported by a network of part-time GP tutors funded by the Department of Health through the Postgraduate Medical and Dental Board. Since their inception in 1981 they have evolved to become 'Quality Circles' engaged in a process of continuous performance improvement through quality assurance.

To further develop this more meaningful CME, those GPs involved will need to give it a higher priority. Every GP should be part of a 'quality circle'. Health care managers and policy makers can support these 'quality circles' by recognising them as a work activity, participation in which would be funded separately from general study leave. The tasks of tutoring, teaching, group leading, and mentoring must also continue to be approached in an increasingly professional way. This in turn will demand a structured approach to training and supporting a 'school' of CME educators. The focus of CME activity should continue to be practice- or locally-based.

GPs must face the challenge of clarifying the role of the pharmaceutical industry in CME. Doctors must be clearly independent of the industry and be seen to be so. Promotion should never be a part of the content of CME programmes and selective funding should not distort the CME agenda. With these provisos, however, the support for much worthwhile CME provided by the pharmaceutical industry should be acknowledged, and GPs should insist that any legislative action to curb sponsorship must be matched with replacement funding.

One special form of CME is distance learning. The recent rapid development of the internet and intranets present new challenges in this field. The ready availability of cheap interactive opportunities not only with the 'education centre' but between participants themselves transforms the isolated nature of this system of learning.

The development of CME as the central activity of quality assurance (QA) is the greatest challenge of all. QA should be an educational activity which forms the largest part of self-directed lifelong learning. We should review our own performance as part of our daily work. We should have the protected time and funding to do so. QA is the best way to define our learning needs.

In many parts of Europe reaccreditation and recertification are being actively debated. The challenge will be to convince representatives of the consumer that a voluntary system of self-regulation is the most effective way of getting doctors to be 'good'.

The obligation to learn is unenforceable. You can force attendance by regulation or financial penalty but you cannot force learning – much less improved competence, performance or patient outcomes. Doctors should be free to choose their own educational activities but with that freedom must also accept a responsibility to assure the public that they are maintaining their competence. The challenge is to put in place a system of self-regulation through quality assurance using optimal guidelines which will satisfy public demand.

At the same time we must acknowledge that for a minority of our colleagues special forms of assessment using minimal guidelines will be required to establish their fitness to practice. Identifying those doctors who need to be specially assessed is difficult and will at times be necessarily arbitrary. Natural justice requires that remedial education programmes be available to rehabilitate those who fail to meet the minimum standard.

AGENDA FOR CHANGE

In summary therefore the challenges facing us suggest the following agenda for change. We must begin by accepting the need for change. In planning for it we must have a new partnership between government, the medical profession, the medical schools and consumer representatives. We must plan in the medium term and try to avoid ad hoc decision making from year to year.

We must look at health care globally and not just at the primary or secondary care sectors as if they were entirely unrelated. If we accept that the appropriate use of specialists requires their services to be accessed through a general practitioner, then we must maintain a defined gatekeeper role. Care should be actively transferred from secondary to primary care, and from primary care to self care. This should be the key priority in health care.

In an ideal world people would use health services effectively. Most of the time this would mean tolerating, alleviating or even curing their self-limiting illnesses using their own medical knowledge, behavioural adjustments and simple remedies available over the counter. Starting in the schools and through the media we must educate the Irish people about health and illness.

Colleges and other academic bodies should develop their advisory role in policy making and effective professional trade unions should defend the interests of their members. These functions should be separate.

General practice must continue to perfect a clear definition of the primary medical generalist and link to it a demand for a balanced medical workforce, particularly with regard to specialist mix. The ratio of generalists to specialists must be maintained at two to one. There must be a national policy on the numbers of doctors, their distribution and retention.

As general practitioners, if we define ourselves in terms of the patients we care for and the continuity of our relationship with them we must call clearly for defined patient lists.

General practitioners should have a role to play within the medical profession in balancing the biotechnical emphasis of specialists by stressing the importance of personal care.

GPs must strive to make our discipline as firmly based on evidence as it can be and wherever possible use rational scientific method when attempting to solve patient problems. However, we must also be realistic. For the foreseeable future most of the time we will not be able to make specific diagnoses and offer specific treatment. We will continue to deal with much undifferentiated illness for which we have only symptomatic or presumptive treatment. The scope of this review has not allowed for an adequate discussion of the challenge of research. What is clear however is that the development of the discipline requires reliable information.

Medical schools must establish mechanisms by which they respond to national needs and aspirations in health care.

Serious investment of time and resources must now be devoted to establish active performance-based systems of CME which include quality assurance. These should form the basis of a voluntary system of recertification for doctors and reaccreditation for practices.

Finally the future of the health service and its cost must be a matter for society at large. Its development requires a balance between policy makers, health care managers, consumers, practitioners and medical teachers. Their consensus must reflect their different priorities. The socio-political perspective as defined by WHO embraces four key elements – relevance, equity, quality and cost effectiveness. The professional emphasis is on excellence, autonomy, responsibility, rationality and ethical standards. Consumers stress access, availability, communication, continuity, problem solving, and shared decision making when appropriate. There is scope for a 'social contract' on health which sets out medium term goals and embraces the priorities of these principal 'stake holders'.

CHAPTER 5

Thoughts on the Acute Hospital System

Sean Conroy

We have arrived at our present acute hospital system along different evolutionary strands dotted with workhouses, charitable infirmaries, county homes and private clinics. This network has been variously funded through donations, poor law rates, central taxation, insurance and user-charges. Various goals have driven the system to where it is now: the need to care for the destitute, the destitute sick, the sick poor, the contagiously infected, mothers and children, the public in general, accident victims, etc. There have been other interests: the preservation of doctors' incomes, the preservation of the power of the churches, the election and re-election of politicians and the provision of employment.

The services provided in hospitals, particularly since the advent of anaesthesia, bacteriology, pathology and radiology, have changed from comfort, containment and palliation to diagnostics, therapeutics and some disease prevention and health promotion. Whereas the workhouse infirmaries delivered care through resident doctors and able-bodied inmates, hospitals are now staffed with dozens of medical, nursing and other caregivers. Governance of hospitals, that is the exercise of trustee ownership, has at various times involved the wealthy, the churches, doctors, politicians, civil servants and representatives from community groups.

It is not known how well hospitals function, given their complexity and the nebulous nature of their 'product'. If, for example, they manufactured televisions, the market place would evaluate; overly expensive and/or poor quality and/or poorly serviced sets would not be bought. Hospitals are in a much more important business; they seek to effect health (and increasingly social) gain. This gain is difficult to measure and the financial cost of the effort involved is difficult to pass judgement on. With the daily advent of new medications, machines, procedures and therapies, hospitals appear capable of absorbing as much money as is thrown at them, without major change in the health of the populations they serve. In addition, the complex, interdisciplinary processes used by hospitals to deliver care are largely unexamined or refined. The perception of a hospital's worth still appears to be largely linked to its bed numbers. There is an emphasis on structure, little on process and, only recently, some on outcome.

Major issues affecting hospitals include:-

- Governance
- Patient focus
- The public-private mix
- The role of doctors
- Assessment and accountability.

These are at the heart of the hospital debate and will have to be addressed if the key principles underlying *Shaping a Healthier Future* – equity, quality and accountability – are to reign.

GOVERNANCE

Governance is the exercise of ownership by a group of people, usually acting in trust for another or others. This is the function of boards. Boards sit atop all hospitals, whether they be the boards of voluntary hospitals or health boards. All activity in a hospital, by all staff including doctors, needs to be focused on the goals enunciated by the board. Governance is of critical importance. Unfortunately, the attention directed to it is in inverse proportion to its importance and it is thus poorly performed. Increasingly, the public will expect boards to listen to them and to be accountable for all of the activity in hospitals, clinical activity included.

The ownership role exercised by boards is given in trust either by the Minister for Health or, for example, by a religious order. The rigid control exercised by the Department of Health in many of the operational affairs is not compatible with good governance, unless it is decided that there is only one board in the country, the cabinet. Further, even with the 1996 accountability legislation, it will never be possible to have accountability ordinarily reside at board level until authority is also seen to reside there.

When, as planned, the voluntary hospitals receive their funding from health boards, further refinement and redefinition of the nature and limits of their governance will be necessary. Health board hospitals will sit uncomfortably beside voluntary hospitals in the proposed restructuring and it may be necessary to give them each a board that will be advisory to the health board, thus showing a kind of parity of esteem. It seems likely that a funder-provider relationship will develop between health boards and their hospital boards.

PATIENT FOCUS

Hospitals are large and complex. Although all staff want to look after their patient-clients as well as possible and would list this as their main goal, hospitals have evolved to suit the people who work in them more than the people they serve. There is a power imbalance; patients are less familiar than their carers with the language, surrounds, routine, natural course of illness and likely consequences of treatment. There is still a significant element of benevolent paternalism in the attitude of hospital staff to their patients.

The challenge for the future is to put the patient at the centre of all activity and see the care process as interdisciplinary teamwork, involving porters, nurses, consultants, attendants, etc., all working to provide care that is consistent but also personalised.

Interdisciplinary patient-focused care will require a major change in the way we think. At present, we tend to sectionalise staff (doctors meet with doctors, nurses with nurses, managers with managers, etc.) and segmentalise care (A&E, ICU, wards, are all treated as independent areas) despite the fact that patients make no such distinction as they receive care and move through a hospital. In the future, it is likely that individual hospital staff will identify as closely with their care team as they do now with the peer groups they belong to by virtue of their training. The transition will be painful and staff fears will need to be recognised. It is inevitable that there will be changes in the power balances amongst professions, developments in the area of skill-mix and a degree of matrix reporting.

The very recruitment and retention of hospital staff will be different in the future. Just as in industry, where change is endemic and security tenuous, hospitals will look to targeted recruitment and limited-term contractual employment. There will be less security but hopefully more energy and innovation. Continuous education will be recognised as an integral part of every job description and primary responsibility for its provision will reside with the employer.

THE PUBLIC-PRIVATE MIX

It is a myth that the only or the main reason for the existence of the public-private mix in healthcare is the unaffordability of universally free (i.e. taxation-based) access. Whilst the Department of Finance may have baulked at the cost implications of the Department of Health White Paper of 1947, this was not the only reason the universal system was not introduced. Successful opposition came from doctors, concerned primarily with loss of private fees, and the

Catholic church, concerned with loss of power and influence on the morality of the Irish people. As recently as the Commission on Health Funding (1989), the issue was again debated with the conclusion that separate access to care for private patients is acceptable as long as access for public patients is reasonable.

It can be contended that there is no private-public mix because the two are immiscible, oil and water, and that 'stirring' merely creates an illusion. Left to their own devices, oil always goes to the top and water to the bottom. If a publican paid her barman by the hour for covering the bar and by the drink for covering the lounge, it would be hard to get served in the bar. There is, of course, no reason a national health service could not remunerate hospital doctors on a fee-per-item basis. Separate access should not mean priority access.

At its worst, the present public-private divide constitutes a kind of caste system. The public caste perceives its care as largesse, the private caste perceives its care as service. Nowhere is this seen to greater effect than in the juxtaposition of news items about waiting list initiatives and advertisements for the VHI depicting a subscriber picking the day he will have his surgery. It often appears that growth in private healthcare is dependent on a poor perception of public healthcare. This is not by way of a conspiracy theory; the present 'mix' quite simply makes some types of behaviour more likely than others. In this regard, waiting lists are weapons and must be decommissioned.

THE ROLE OF DOCTORS

Irish doctors and the Irish medical schools have contributed to the body of medical science and to the history of the medical profession out of all proportion to their numbers. Great men and women have done and continue to do great work. There is a downside, however. Many of the utterances of their leaders and representatives would suggest that improvements in public health depend on unfettered and full-blooded private practice of whatever range and volume they deem appropriate. Because of the historical absence of consumerism, doctors often capture the advocacy role, even when it is self-interest that is speaking.

Clinical autonomy is important to all doctors and their patients but it is most often cited as a reason not to be held accountable by boards for the quality of medical care or the judicious use of resources, and as a reason not to form structured medical staff organisations. The logic is not easy to follow. Doctors are surely accountable to their patients; and their patients surely expect hospital and health board governing bodies to be in charge of their organisations. Current methods of consultant appointment do little to foster a climate conducive to the changes needed; consultants function as independent practitioners instead of independent contractors.

Ireland produces four times as many doctors per capita as Canada and yet a very large proportion of non-consultant hospital doctors (NCHDs) are not from Ireland, not even from the EU. Why is this? Some consultants will argue that there is no problem; Irish doctors have always gone abroad to train and then come back to enrich Irish healthcare with the benefits of their learning and experience. If this is so, we should by now be in a position to train to an excellent level any young doctor who wishes to become a consultant, with perhaps the occasional six months or so structured placement abroad. Surely the educators of NCHDs should be united into one coherent body and surely the deciding factor in placing an NCHD with a consultant should be the educational advantage achieved as opposed to the service need fulfilled. When this happens, there will be more consultants and fewer NCHDs and the meaning of the word consultant will change.

ASSESSMENT & ACCOUNTABILITY

Donabedian, the father of modern academic quality assessment in health, described it as an 'exasperatingly complex subject'. In the last 20 years, the 'quality movement' has become in some ways an industry, in others a religion. Those in hospitals anxious to compile and act on a 'quality' agenda can be forgiven if moidered (it seems the only word appropriate) by the profusion of approaches and concepts; QA (quality assurance), QM (quality management), CQI (continuous quality improvement), TQM (total quality management), outcomes, best practice, clinical guidelines, process re-engineering, etc. Everyone now has some familiarity with the trilogy of structure, process and outcome. Because of the rapid pace of change in thinking about quality, hospital staff enthused about the subject often fear that the approach they choose will be pronounced obsolete just as they become familiar with it, in the same way that last year's revolutionary personal computer is this year's paperweight. Perhaps it is best to abandon the jargon and the fads and look at the basic changes in the healthcare climate that are causing the increased emphasis on 'quality', particularly as it applies to hospitals.

–   Healthcare consumerism is arriving. A combination of recent relative wealth, increasing levels of education and a heightened awareness of other nations and other ways of doing things has altered Irish society from a tradition characterised by inertia and obedience to a new era characterised by change and questioning. Amongst old untouchables feeling this shift are religion and medicine/healthcare. In the latter arena, hospitals are highly visible.

–   Government is evolving a more business-like approach in response to a variety of pressures, including the increased sophistication of the electorate, the demands of membership of the EU and the acceptance that there is no inherent contradiction in using the methodologies of private enterprise to achieve agreed social goals. Witness the change from a policy of increased employment in the public sector and anonymity of civil servants to the strategic management initiative, accountability legislation, value for money, etc. The Department of Finance now wants to know what it is buying with the health allocation. Hospitals are expensive.

–   Developments within healthcare have also created a critical climate. The increased awareness of, investment in and preference for community-based care have created scrutiny of the resources put into hospitals, particularly given the apparent never-ending increase in the expensive high technology demands they express. The non-hospital sector seems now to relentlessly identify need, quantify desired intervention and measure results, activities and skills that successfully capture resources. A significant feature of community development is the increasing role of non-medical professionals who, understandably, enjoy the freedom from medical domination associated with traditional institution-based care. Hospitals, traditionally given the lion's share of funds on the simple basis of 'activity', often despite any obvious internal consensus between medical specialities or between consultants and management, now find the going tougher.

–   The existence of the public-private mix has resulted in the perception of a two-tier system. Implicit in this is the belief by many, if not most that public care is inferior. Thus there is an interest, even if morbid, in what this difference is. To measure the difference, we have to measure.

In the hospital sector, the new era will be one of assessment and accountability. These two words can suffice, without recourse to the quality jargon. The emphasis will be on understanding the health and social status of the population, those aspects that need improvement, those that can be improved, what measurable contribution hospitals can make to this endeavour and at what price. Since this approach starts by looking at the community, it follows that each hospital will need to have a clear sense of its strategic position in healthcare and a much increased awareness of the interdependence of its staff and the fact that their goals are shared. Monitoring the achievement of these goals will produce a climate in which staff will pick various 'quality' tools and methods because they look like they'll do the job, rather than grabbing them first and then wondering what job they do. The recently established departments of public health have an opportunity to help staff to ask the right questions of themselves and their patients.

There is also a lot to be gained by the introduction of an accreditation system like the Canadian Council for Health Services Accreditation. At its best, a hospital being surveyed under such a system is invigorated and enlivened by the experience of being visited and surveyed by a team of peers who help staff to look at themselves and at how well they are living up to agreed standards. Accreditation can change hospital culture and promote openness to new ideas, an interdisciplinary approach to care, patient focus, a climate of continuing education and an awareness of the nature and importance of governance, all readily identifiable issues facing Irish hospitals.

CONCLUSION

Perhaps the future for hospitals, as the Department of Health enters its second half-century, is not 'physician, heal thyself', but rather 'hospital, assess thyself'. It won't be boring.

CHAPTER 6

Child Welfare

Owen Keenan

INTRODUCTION

Considering the extent of contemporary public and media interest in issues relating to children for which the Department of Health has responsibility, it is worth noting that the Department's functions in this area are of relatively recent origin. At the time of its establishment in 1947 the Department's concern with regard to children related to the protection of child health through services administered in each area by the local authority. Child welfare as we understand it to-day is a much broader concept encompassing the social, emotional, educational and economic aspects of well-being in addition to the needs of vulnerable children for care and protection. With the establishment of the health boards in 1970 it was envisaged that their community-based personal social services would adopt an integrated approach to advancing the welfare of various groups within the community, for example the elderly, people with disabilities, children, etc., similar to the model which was at that time in the process of being adopted in England and Wales following the Seebohm proposals for the reorganisation of social services. In the event, delays in the resourcing and recruitment of social workers quickly resulted in the effective concentration of this service on referrals concerning children and families.

Coinciding, as it did, with developing international awareness and concepts relating to 'battered child syndrome', the health boards' social work services soon developed a child protection perspective which, prior to their advent, had been the administrative responsibility of the Irish Society for the Prevention of Cruelty to Children from 1956 and, previously, of its United Kingdom-based parent organisation, the National Society for the Prevention of Cruelty to Children. Children in care were generally placed in large orphanages and residential centres usually managed by religious orders. These came under the responsibility of the Department of Education and this continued for some time after the establishment of the health boards.

There was at this time a gathering impetus for change and reform. The publication in 1966 of *Some of Our Children*, a report by the Tuairim study group, had led to the appointment in 1968 by the Minister for Education of the Kennedy Committee to review the state of the country's industrial schools and reformatories. The Kennedy Report, published in 1970, made far-reaching recommendations for reform and advised that the Department of Health should have overall responsibility for all child care services. This accorded with the demands of CARE – the Campaign for the Care of Deprived Children – which was an influential lobbying group in the 1970s and 1980s.

In 1974 the Government decided to assign primary responsibility for child care to the Minister for Health. The Minister, Brendan Corish TD, established the Task Force on Child Care Services to make recommendations on the extension and improvement of services for deprived children and to prepare a child care bill. The Task Force reported in 1980 and made an extensive number of recommendations for the reform of the child care services. It did not, however, include a draft child care bill. The Report urged that the priority of the services should be the provision of support to enable children to remain within their families; endorsed the integration of child care services under the Minister for Health; and made a series of recommendations which would amount, if implemented, to a radical restructuring of the child care system.

The Department of Health assumed responsibility for residential care facilities, other than for residential special schools, from the Department of Education in 1982. Funding for residential homes changed from a capitation system to a budget basis in 1984. The Department of Health also acquired responsibility for adoption around this time. The first adoption legislation had been passed in 1952, providing for the regulation of a legal adoption system under an Adoption Board which was established on 1 January 1953. Responsibility for adoption was assigned to the Minister for Justice. Thirty years later, on 1 January 1983, this responsibility was transferred to the Minister for Health, Barry Desmond TD, who established a Review Committee on Adoption Services in April 1983. This reported in May 1984. Only a few of its recommendations have been implemented.

REPORT OF TASK FORCE

By the time the Task Force Report was published in 1981, a number of factors had come into play which were to seriously restrict progress on the updating of the child care system for a decade. They included three governments within a period of eighteen months and, of greater significance, the fact that by the early 1980s the Irish economy was in serious difficulty. The development and expansion of the child care system was not considered viable at this time although it should be acknowledged that it was recognised as a priority which should be planned for in the expectation that the economy would eventually improve.

The fact that the Task Force Report itself presented difficulties should also be acknowledged. Undoubtedly a most important report, which continues to be largely relevant, in the seven years it took from beginning to end much of the momentum which had led to its establishment in the first place was dissipated. Furthermore it consisted of both a majority and a supplementary report, the latter written by those members of the Task Force who were not civil servants. The extensive Supplementary Report dealt with matters of policy, structure and service not supported by the majority and also included comprehensive consideration of, and recommendations concerning, the adoption services, which were judged by the majority of members to be outside their terms of reference. In a favourable political and economic climate it would have taken considerable skill and determination to reconcile such diversity of opinion into coherent and progressive draft legislation. In the event other priorities were adopted and much of the zeal and enthusiasm for reform of the child care system was lost. Although the introduction of new child care legislation remained a declared priority of government, it was to be a further four years before the Child (Care and Protection) Bill 1985 was published. It was subsequently superseded, following a further change of government, by the Child Care Bill 1988. This bill was eventually passed by the Oireachtas, with amendments, and was signed into law in July 1991.

The main features of the Child Care Act 1991 are the assignment of responsibility to health boards for the promotion of the welfare of children (up to the age of 18 years) who are not receiving adequate care and protection; provision for the protection of children in emergencies; care proceedings including the introduction of supervision orders; responsibilities of health boards for children in care; for the supervision of pre-school services; and for the regulation of children's residential centres. A clear line may be traced from the publication of the Tuairim Report in 1966 to the eventual passing of the 1991 legislation. There had been many significant milestones along the way but, in spite of a gestation period lasting a quarter of a century, more than a further five years was to elapse before the Child Care Act 1991 was fully implemented in December 1996.

Nor did the government of the day apparently feel compelled to implement the new legislation more hastily. The *Programme for Economic and Social Progress* (PESP) which represented the framework for action agreed by the government and social partners in 1991 actually stated that the Act would be implemented on a phased basis over seven years. An additional £1m was provided from National Lottery funds in 1991 to cover the costs of the initial phase. The primary legislation concerning children at that time was still the Children Act 1908, passed under British administration, and the protracted and unacceptable delay over two and a half decades in producing the new legislation led this writer to describe child care, in 1991, as 'the most neglected area of public policy since the foundation of the State' (Keenan, 1991). A further £2m from National Lottery funds was allocated in 1992. In spite of commitments given, no additional provision was made by the new government in the January 1993 Budget to allow for the further implementation of the legislation. However, 1993 was to prove a watershed in the development of Ireland's provision for children at risk.

KILKENNY INCEST CASE

In March 1993, having previously pleaded guilty to six specimen charges involving rape, incest and assault, a man was sentenced in the Central Criminal Court to a total of seven years penal servitude. The charges related to persistent incest involving his daughter over a period of sixteen years. The family had been known to the relevant health board and other statutory agencies over many years. In what became known as the Kilkenny Incest Case, a great deal of media comment centred on the health board's perceived failure to intervene effectively to end this abuse. The Minister for Health, Brendan Howlin TD, quickly established an inquiry which reported within two months.

On the publication of the Kilkenny Incest Inquiry Report in May 1993 the Minister for Health announced: that the government had provided a total of £35m phased over three years to support the full implementation of the Child Care Act 1991; that new protocols were to be established to guide collaboration between health boards and the Garda Siochána in relation to children at risk; and that he was establishing a Child Care Policy Unit within the Department of Health. Over the subsequent three years the additional resources have had a significant impact on the level of child care provision, most notably a major increase in the number of social workers and other child care personnel employed, the expansion and development of residential care and the establishment of a number of family support services.

A further consequence of the Kilkenny Incest Case has been heightened public awareness of and concern for children at risk – largely arising from a sustained high level of media interest in the issue. It is not overstating the case to suggest that child abuse has been one of the most prominent matters of public and media interest of the 1990s to date. As a result a number of other cases involving both individual and institutional abuse of children has come to light and influenced the continuing development of the child care systems. Perhaps most dramatically matters concerning how child abuse issues are treated and, specifically, delays in the Attorney General's Office in handling a paedophilia case led directly to the fall of the Fianna Fáil/Labour Coalition Government in November 1994.

The appointment by the subsequent coalition government of a minister of state with special responsibility for children at the Departments of Health, Education and Justice was an unique departure from previous practice and was designed to strengthen the integration of all relevant parts of the child care system. The Minister appointed, Austin Currie TD, was assigned specific responsibility for the implementation of the Child Care Act 1991, the preparation of new juvenile justice legislation and the effective co-ordination of the child care policies and provisions of the three Departments. The creation of an office of Minister for Children attracted international interest as it is markedly rare for governments to make such appointments at either senior or junior ministerial rank. At the time of writing it is premature to make a comprehensive and objective assessment of the success or otherwise of this appointment, but the positive features undoubtedly include the benefit of having a specific focus on child care matters. The evidence suggests, however, that there are matters of policy, resources and structure that are even more critical to the successful development of the child care system than the specific assignment of political responsibility.

It must be said that in terms of legislation, resources, staffing, services, protocols, and political, media and public attention, the challenge of protecting children in Ireland and promoting their welfare has been advanced to a greater extent in the present decade than at any time in the previous seventy years. Yet paradoxically many Irish children are currently faced with greater problems than ever before. Meanwhile the system which has been constructed to support and protect them faces unprecedented levels of demand, and the expectations of politicians, media and public. This combination of factors has the potential to spiral out of control.

NEED FOR ADEQUATE RESOURCES

Had the resources provided for our child care services been consistently increased over a lengthy period of years, it is possible that in time a stage would have been reached where a reasonably adequate response to children who were vulnerable might have been expected. Unfortunately this has never been the case. We have seen the tortuous progress that was made towards the preparation and enactment of the Child Care Act 1991, and reference has been made to the resourcing difficulties especially encountered during the 1980s. Yet while resource provision was standing still or being reduced in real terms, health board child care services were experiencing significantly increased levels of need and demand, coupled with ever-greater expectations of their capacity to protect children at risk. For example, the number of cases of suspected child abuse reported to health boards doubled between 1987 and 1989, as did the number of confirmed cases.

The demands on health boards have continued to increase. The provision of substantially increased funding following the publication of the Kilkenny Report in May 1993 was intended to facilitate the health boards in making a more adequate and effective response to the reports they were receiving concerning children at risk. The impact of the additional resources may be seen in the substantial increase in social work, child care and other professional posts within health boards. New management posts and structures have been established; an investment has been made in improving the quality of residential care; additional residential places have been created, particularly in specialised units and emergency accommodation, for example in hostels and refuges; an emergency night and weekend social work service has been established in Dublin; some additional family support services have been established.

INCREASED REPORTING OF CHILD ABUSE

The emphasis in the deployment of the additional resources has been heavily weighted towards the development of health boards' capacity to intervene, investigate and provide a response to extreme cases of child abuse, family dysfunction or breakdown and crisis situations. Whilst necessary, given the prior failure to construct an effective and resourced child protection infrastructure, the recent development has resulted in improving the quality of the system's response to emergency situations but has had little impact on the level of need or demand. On the contrary, the heightened awareness of both the public and professionals has led to a further substantial increase in the number of child abuse referrals to health boards, which increased by 25% each year between 1993 and 1995. In fact there was a fourfold increase in the number of child abuse referrals to health boards between 1987 and 1995, while the number of confirmed cases trebled in the same period. Thus the additional capacity afforded to health boards following the publication of the Kilkenny Report has been largely absorbed by the increase in demand.

The increased reporting of suspected or actual child abuse should be attributed to the heightened recognition of the fact of child abuse and awareness of its symptoms, rather than to suggest a commensurate increase in its incidence over this period. Indeed some satisfaction can be taken from the fact that children who are being abused, exploited or neglected are now much more likely to come to the attention of the appropriate authorities than was the case heretofore. Nevertheless Irish child abuse prevalence rates continue to be historically lower than international rates. It is the concern to fully realise the system's capacity to identify all cases of children at risk – irrespective of the attendant complexities of its implementation – which has led to calls for the introduction of mandatory reporting. In declaring my personal conviction that mandatory reporting should be introduced it is important that I acknowledge that the opposing view is held by many with equal sincerity and integrity. The constraints of this essay do not allow me to expand on the relevant arguments. The core issue, though, must be the aspiration to take every reasonable step to identify and respond effectively to every child at risk, rather than to seek to limit demand to the capacity of the system.

NEED FOR GREATER COMMITMENT

The fact must be faced that Ireland's provision for vulnerable children has been seriously deficient and has never reached the level of sophistication that it could, or should, have done. Whether for political, sociological or cultural reasons we have never acknowledged the full extent of child care need in the country. While recognising the advances that have been made in recent times, the fact is that developments have been slow, reactive and piecemeal. There has been no sense of vision, urgency or idealism. This is evident in the lengthy gestation of our current legislation; the fact that it was 1979 (the International Year of the Child) before the Department of Health established a small Child Care Division; statistics on child abuse only began to be collected in 1983 and continue to be unsatisfactory; and the main impetus for change in the 1990s has been largely driven by media attention rather than by a proactive concern to realise a positive vision for children.

Perhaps the most significant implication of the media interest has been the exposure of failure in the system to date. Any organism will move to defend itself against perceived attack and it is no surprise when the child protection system reacts to criticism in this way. The consequence however is that a system which has never articulated its core objective is, by default, in danger of establishing the prevention of child abuse as its primary task. It is doomed to fail.

It is possible to reduce the incidence of child abuse. It is also possible to improve professionals' skills in recognising individuals and families that are pathologically dangerous. It is possible to identify early and intervene effectively in specific cases of child abuse. It is not possible, however, to prevent child abuse occurring in total and it is unfortunately inevitable that some children will be severely, perhaps fatally, abused. A system which denies this reality is both misconceived and itself dangerous. It is essential that we manage the apparent paradox of doing more to protect children whilst accepting the certainty that the system will fail in some cases.

PROMOTING CHILD WELFARE

Prior to the identification of what was then termed non-accidental injury (NAI) following the British Maria Colwell case in the mid-1970s, the thrust of the public child care system was to promote the welfare of children. As awareness of child abuse increased and concern grew, the focus of the child care system narrowed from broad issues of child welfare to the more specific area of protection from physical, sexual and emotional abuse and neglect. Indeed whereas physical abuse was the primary concern in the 1970s, sexual abuse has been the subject of growing concern. The danger here is that one finds what one expects to find and a narrow focus can have the effect of excluding everything else. For example, recent child abuse statistics indicate a higher prevalence of sexual abuse relative to emotional abuse and neglect, and in some health board areas sexual abuse is now recorded as the most dominant form of child abuse. Such data should be treated with caution.

There is an urgent need to return to the concept of promoting child welfare as the foundation of our provision for children. It is a broad concept, one which places the well-being of children in all its facets at its core. With the final implementation in full of the Child Care Act 1991, which gives to health boards statutory responsibility for the identification of children in their area who are in need of support and protection, there is an opportunity to return to a fuller understanding of the factors that promote children's welfare.

In particular there is a need to acknowledge the benefit and potential for further development of family support services. Comprising a range of specific services such as day care centres, family counselling, development of parenting skills, toy libraries, and so on, family support services typically are locally based, involve parents and children together and emphasise prevention and early intervention. They are cost effective, as they provide solutions to problems or potential problems before they have become acute and expensive to reverse. Even more importantly, they contain the human costs of such problems. The history of recent years as we have invested in the development of our capacity to protect children has demonstrated, however, that preventive measures, however worthy, cannot equitably compete for resources with crisis or emergency demands. If we are to have serious intent which values the preventive approach, specific budgets will need to be created and protected, as resources will otherwise be continually siphoned off to meet more urgent demands. An effective preventive strategy will have significant implications for the system as a whole and will demand the integration of the resources and capacities of a number of key sectors and affect how these are organised and function.

There is a clear, proven correlation between social deprivation, educational disadvantage, poverty, unstable relationships, poor health and housing, addiction, crime, etc, yet we have failed so far to integrate this knowledge into the way we structure and deliver responses to these social concerns. The way public services are structured and ordered continues to have a disproportionate influence over the quality and cohesion of their delivery. As a result the strategies of one part of the system can be undone by the actions of another. In relation to child care there have been repeated calls for the disparate parts of the system to be gathered together under the responsibility of a single Department for Children. In spite of its merits the proposal has fundamental flaws. At what point, for example, would the line be drawn between child and adult education? Who would investigate crimes committed against/by children? How would child welfare and family welfare interventions be differentiated?

NEED FOR GREATER INTEGRATION

Indeed the resolution of difficulties caused by fragmentation has more to do with clarity of purpose and objectives than it does with structures. Clearly more effective outcomes for children could be achieved if a greater degree of integration was established both within individual health boards, and between health boards and other bodies of relevance to the sector.

Within health board community care departments, the professional staffing model devised when they were established in the early 1970s is still effectively intact but is to-day under severe pressure due to major expansion, both of staff and need. The various disciplines are grouped, supervised and managed as discrete entities. This has promoted identification with one's immediate professional colleagues to the detriment of inter-disciplinary confidence and collaboration. These divisions have frequently been reinforced by separateness of premises, location and resource provision. As a result legitimate differences of task and perspective have too often led to rivalries rather than to resolution and accommodation. Related difficulties have also been known to exist within health boards between, for example, community care personnel, child psychiatric services and general hospitals.

There is now an urgency about modelling new approaches to professional practice, based on encouraging more integrative and collaborative strategies, piloting innovative supervision and accountability initiatives and giving emphasis to the actual benefits for children and their families. Such approaches, if they are to be effective, will also require the committed support of health board managements. Frontline staff need to be supported in the pursuit of the attainable, particularly in the promotion of the welfare of children, while the limitations and constraints of their role also need to be acknowledged and accepted.

There is also a need to consider how the initiatives and responsibilities of various bodies, both statutory and voluntary, in supporting child and family welfare at community level might be better integrated. The potential here ranges from ensuring consistency between the policies and practices of each body, to maximising the accessibility of services, for example by sharing premises. One would hope that this would result in greater coherence in the respective pre-school provision of health boards and the Department of Education and the maximising of the availability of public buildings in each community.

THE CONSUMER VOICE

In extending our capacity to effectively support the welfare of children and families at community level two further developments are of particular importance. Firstly there is the acknowledgement of the relevance, importance and effectiveness of the consumer voice. The perspectives and experiences of families have a richness and a relevance for service providers which cannot be obtained from any other source. Secondly there is Ireland's ratification of the United Nations Convention on the Rights of the Child. If this is to be meaningfully implemented it must be central to the child welfare system. Article 12 of the Convention refers to the right of children to be consulted on all matters of relevance to them. This has particular significance for children in care or who may be subject to the intervention of the child care system. It is essential that the centrality and relevance of the participation of children and their families be fully embraced.

This also symbolises an acknowledgement of the interrelationship between the private and public dimensions of child care need. Certainly a significant number of children experience difficulties due to their families' pathologies, and there are families which are inherently dangerous and require a specific type of intervention. In the main, however, most of the problems experienced by children have a public or social policy aspect, for example, poverty, unemployment, crime, etc. An approach which encompasses the frequently hard-edged and experienced perspective of the consumer is the most effective means of understanding their problems and correcting such policies. Besides, while it might be more comforting to interpret the range of difficulties that a significant number of children encounter as, effectively, the fault of their parents, this denies the reality of the negative impact of many public policies on certain groups, and also of structural inequities within society.

LOOKING TO THE FUTURE

In spite of past neglect and present need there exists to-day, because of both a maturing professional expertise and national economic health, an unique opportunity to construct a much more favourable and equitable future for our children. That future cannot be delivered by the Department of Health in isolation. It can only be realised through adopting a comprehensive and progressive programme of action over a number of years and involving many disparate bodies and groups. If it is to have any prospect of success it must be accompanied by two ingredients that have not been sufficiently evident to-date.

The first is vision. We have not articulated any national aspiration for our children. To what end are the various government departments which have a responsibility for children working? Are they consistent and complementary? What interim targets have been set? How is progress being evaluated? How will we know we have realised our objectives? Effectively, how is our aspiration driving our actions?

The second is commitment, particularly political commitment. Without apportioning blame for past failures, it has to be acknowledged that state provision to promote the welfare of children has not developed as it should. Certainly there have been improvements in recent years, for example in strengthening the child protection system, and attempts to target educational disadvantage. Yet already there are worrying signs of a view emerging that the additional investment of recent years is sufficient and that it is now time to address the needs of other target groups. This is not supported by the facts, which show that we have begun to construct an effective system but have not yet succeeded in reducing the pressure on existing services. It is redolent of either complacency or indifference. Complacency, that everything is now satisfactory; or indifference, that enough has now been done and we have achieved a level of child care need that is acceptable. Either of these perspectives is misguided and dangerous. Without the will no progress is attainable. Commitment may be weakened by concern about a possible never-ending demand for additional resources. In this regard it should be borne in mind that :

* the formulation of a concerted programme of action towards a shared goal will reduce duplication, deliver more effective outcomes, and give a better return on existing expenditures;

* a shift from emergency provision to increased emphasis on preventive measures will result in better outcomes in both human terms and cost effectiveness;

* the decline in the birth rate offers the opportunity to target the savings accruing towards those children and families in greatest need. To maximise this opportunity, new levels of budget flexibility between departments and other bodies will have to be achieved;

* increasing experience of the benefits of engaging service users and communities through involving them meaningfully in the process of advancing the welfare of children offers the opportunity for more effective strategies to be devised and implemented.

Let us not ignore, however, the fact that additional resources will be necessary over several years if the situation of children in Ireland, which in many respects continues to worsen, is to be reversed. In total budgetary terms the resources required are relatively modest and can be fully justified in terms of future human and economic benefits to society. This is a political, ultimately public, choice.

Essentially there is a need for Ireland to articulate a vision of how it might aspire to provide for its children in the future. For example it might assert a determination to eliminate child poverty, to ensure that no young person would be without suitable accommodation or excluded from school, and that no child in need would be denied protection due to lack of appropriate resources. Recognising that the current situation falls far short of such an aspiration, it could only be realised in the long term. Since it would take longer than the lifetime of a single government, say ten years, it would be necessary to achieve broad all-party support and commitment to pursue it, although it has to be recognised that individual parties might approach its implementation differently. A national plan to support the realisation of the aspiration would need to be prepared. This would have to be specific about interim priorities and targets and evaluation of progress. Finally, a structure would need to be established to ensure that all necessary components were harnessed and directed towards the achievement of both interim and ultimate objectives. This would be the 'engine' to drive action. It would not necessarily have to be a large body, but it would need to have real political and administrative clout. Existing proposals for a National Children's Council or a Child Care Authority could be considered for this role. The main imperative would be its capacity to deliver – this would require authority, independence, the capacity to communicate directly with the public, and access to political power.

This may well be regarded as rational, but unrealistic. It is certainly idealistic to aspire to the elimination of child poverty and the provision of more appropriate responses to children experiencing abuse and serious deprivations. It is also easy to acknowledge the challenges of achieving effective collaboration among a substantial number of bodies including the voluntary sector, a prerequisite for real progress. The requirement for flexibility in sharing and transferring resources between government departments would be particularly formidable. Yet the story so far suggests that we need a new paradigm. It is usual for the unfamiliar to be uncomfortable and the object of some resistance. There is, nevertheless, substantial concern and commitment in the system for the welfare of children which, cemented by the pursuit of a common objective and with firm political drive and determination, offers potential for real progress. Such an integrated approach also has the benefit of relieving any one part of the system of expectations which it cannot possibly deliver. For example, in recent years the Department of Health's responsibilities for child care have rated amongst its most politically sensitive functions yet, arguably, the one that is least amenable to its direct intervention. It is, in fact, only by playing its part in supporting the welfare of children as a whole that the interests of protecting children can best, if incompletely, be achieved.

The way a society provides for its children suggests much about its compassion, values and economic well-being but it says perhaps more about its confidence in its future. Confidence is not a word that springs easily to mind in considering Ireland's social development since independence. Yet, at a time when more favourable winds have begun to blow, confidence combined with determination could substantially alter the way we provide for our children's welfare. Certainly a positive, progressive and properly resourced commitment to children is an investment that will pay back dividends to society.

CHAPTER 7

The Development of a Health Policy for Women

Evelyn Mahon

In this chapter I will review the major changes in women's lives over the last fifty years. During the period under consideration Ireland changed from a very traditional rural based society into a modern society. In traditional society individual needs are subordinated to those of kinship and the maintenance of the social system. Modern society, however, is characterised by increased individualism wherein the self becomes a reflexive project, continually examining itself and changing over time. Practices in traditional society encouraged a fatalistic orientation towards the future, while modernity promotes activism which leads one to acquire a new sense of self. Subjects like psychology and sociology, modes of therapies and counselling of all kinds help in the reflexivity of the self. As Giddens describes it: 'modernity . . . breaks down the protective framework of the small community and of tradition, replacing these with much larger impersonal organizations' (Giddens, 1991, 33). Therapy is 'an expression of the reflexivity of the self – a phenomenon which, on the level of the individual, like the broader institutions of modernity, balances opportunity and potential catastrophe in equal measure' (Giddens, 1991, 34). These changes from traditional to modern society are reflected in the activities of the Department of Health over the last fifty years. It is this progression from traditionalism to modernism that I will examine, focusing on specific areas of women's health, namely: life expectancy, family planning and health behaviour.

THE LIFE EXPECTANCY OF WOMEN

One might first ask, what has the Department of Health achieved for women since its inception in 1947? Firstly, it has made a contribution to the social and scientific advances which have led to the considerable increase in women's life expectancy – from 67 years in 1950-52 to 77.9 in 1992. Early in this century Ireland was unique in Europe in having higher male than female survival rates at any age (Coleman, 1992, 69). This deviant pattern persisted until the 1930s. In 1950-52, the difference in Ireland between men and women's life expectancy was still very small: 64.5 for men as contrasted with 67.1 for women. Some commentators have used this statistic as an indicator of the extent to which women were systematically disadvantaged in Ireland. Thus recent gains in the life expectancy of women are deemed a reflection of the erosion of disadvantage (Pyle, 1990; Fitzpatrick, 1984)[1].

This increased life expectancy can be attributed to three factors: nutrition, public hygiene and contraception. While the first two factors have an impact on both men and women, the latter is woman-specific; the benefits of contraception accrue primarily to women.

A second very important indicator of women's well-being is the number of maternal deaths per live births. In 1947 the number of deaths was 148[2]; this declined to eight in 1983 and there were no maternal deaths in 1993. Improved pre-natal and maternity care and access to family planning have contributed to this decline. There has also been a decline in the number of higher order births. The percentage of births to mothers having their first pregnancy has increased from 20.2% in 1957, to 28.6% in 1981 and to 35.4% in 1993. Births to mothers with four or more children declined from 14.8% in 1981, to 8.2% in 1993.

This change in fertility patterns was accomplished in Ireland much later than in other European states. While most European countries began to adopt family planning within marriage from the 1870s onwards, this was not the case in Ireland (Coleman, 1992, 59).

The 1957 report on vital statistics noted that Irish women married later than those in England and Wales, had a larger number of children and continued to bear children for a greater number of years. In that year, 40% of all births in England and Wales were first births, as contrasted with only 21% of births in Ireland. As regards parity, 19% of births in Ireland were 6th to 10th order births as contrasted with only 3.9% in England. The exceptional nature of Irish demographic patterns among European countries has been of interest to demographers who tried to ascertain why traditional fertility patterns persisted in Ireland. Part of the answer certainly can be found in the history of the development of family planning policies in the Department of Health.

From its inception the Department of Health, like all departments, had to carve out its role within the social and political fabric of its time. The formation of state policy in all areas from the nineteen-thirties onwards was influenced by the Catholic church's principle of state subsidiarity. The church opposed excessive state control which it legitimated in terms of opposition to state communism. Instead, the formation of voluntary associations, groups and organisations, as outlined in the papal encyclical *Quadragesimo Anno* (1931), was promoted. Given the status, power, and leadership exercised by the church, many of these organizations became church-dominated ones.

While subsidiarity was the principle of opposition to state interference, the church also feared the introduction of health services which were available in other countries, notably Northern Ireland and the UK, but which were not in accordance with church teaching.

A 1930 encyclical on Christian marriage, *Casti Connubii*, warned against divorce, contraception and abortion and argued that the family was the foundation of moral and social order (Barrington, 1987, 144). This document provided the Irish Catholic hierarchy with a policy document in these areas. It sought to protect its flock from the dissemination of ideas which were contrary to its teaching. It did this by lobbying for the introduction of protective legislation and by curtailing the remit of the Department of Health. In response to the hierarchy's demand for legislative change, the government passed the Censorship of Publications Act in 1929, making it unlawful to print or publish 'any indecent medical, surgical or physiological details the publication of which would be calculated to injure public morals' (Hogan & Whyte, 1994, 947). This included information on contraception and abortion. The Criminal Law (Amendment) Act 1935 prohibited the importation and sale of contraceptives. Catholic social teaching on marriage and divorce was incorporated into the 1937 Constitution.

The 1947 vital statistics reveal some of the issues that the embryonic department had to address. The infant mortality rate was 68 per 1,000 births as contrasted with 41 per 1,000 in England and Wales. Among legitimate infants the mortality rate was 63 per 1000 but among illegitimate births it was 220 per 1000. Tuberculosis (3,700 deaths), cancer (3,962), strokes (3,024) and heart disease (11,118) were the major killers. 130 deaths were due to puerperal causes. Many died from measles, influenza, whooping cough and diphtheria. The effective control of infectious diseases and health promotion required state action and agencies. The new department had to establish its remit and then formulate and implement a health policy, catering both to the physical needs of the mother and her children and to the moral demands of the church.

CHURCH-STATE CONFLICTS

In practice, policy was developed in the context of church-state negotiations and shared responsibilities between statutory and voluntary organisations, a form of Catholic corporatism. It was inevitable that this would also generate conflicts between church authority and state responsibility.

The formation of voluntary and communal organizations to help the poor and the sick was energetically encouraged by Dr John Charles McQuaid, who was appointed Archbishop of Dublin in 1940 (Barrington, 1987, 145). He was ably assisted by Dr Michael Browne, Bishop of Galway, who chaired the Church Commission to examine vocational organisation. The Commission's report emphasised the dangers of bureaucracy. Subsequently the church produced a health policy. This activity placed the newly-appointed Minister for Health in a reactive role, as the church saw itself as having a clear mandate to formulate policy. The development of departments of health and education is therefore best understood within the origins of Catholic vocationalism. It was inevitable that this would lead to a series of church-state conflicts.

The first example of church-state conflict was the Public Health Bill of 1945. This Bill sought to empower county and county boroughs to provide maternity and child health services and to medically inspect all school children. The aim was to provide a unified, free service, which would give continuous care to mothers and children during the ante-natal period, at birth, and until the child reached 16 years of age. It proposed giving explicit powers to local authorities and to educate mothers, and children, in matters relating to health.

However, this proposal was opposed by the church. It argued that compulsory medical inspection was a serious infringement of the natural rights of parents and that the medical inspection of adolescent girls was undesirable. Alarmed at the impact of the provision of free ante-natal and maternity services on their incomes, the Irish Medical Association joined forces with the church in opposing the Bill. The Association's chief protagonist was Dr McPolin, who objected on three bases. First, he stated that the relationship with a doctor could only be guaranteed where the doctor was an independent contractor and the family paid for the services received. Secondly, a free medical service undermined the role of the family because it interfered with the duty of parents to provide for the physical welfare of their children. Thirdly, he argued that the state did not have a role to educate mothers and children – that was the role of the family doctor in conjunction with the church which was the arbitrator of matters of faith and morals. Barrington (1987) argues that McPolin translated genuine medical questions into moral objections to state-controlled medicine. This appealed to the Irish hierarchy and to conservative members of the Irish public.

The first Minister for Health was appointed in January 1947. He counteracted McPolin's arguments, gradually gaining public acceptance for the Bill. However, in October 1947 the Catholic hierarchy privately protested to the government about the new Health Bill. Its objections were put in the context that the Health Act would infringe the rights of individuals, the family, the professions and voluntary institutions. It objected to the danger posed to the morals of women and children by health education. The hierarchy's real fear was it would expose women to information on contraception and abortion, and children to sex education (Barrington, 1987, 187). In addition the hierarchy feared for the future of their control of the voluntary hospitals; they had a vested interest in resisting state control.

Conflict on the Health Act, 1947 continued and its constitutionality was examined. In 1948 there was a general election and a coalition government was formed. A new Minister for Health, Noel Browne, was appointed in 1948. He outlined the broad parameters of the way in which the provision of medical care, enabled by a section of the 1947 Act, would be carried out. However, relations between the medical professions, the church and the minister rapidly deteriorated. The church vigorously objected to the state's role in educating mothers and children and suggested instead that the enabling section of the Health Act, 1947 be amended. Brown was forced to resign and, in the subsequent general election of 1951, health services became a major issue. The coalition parties lost and a victorious Fianna Fáil government promised to extend the health services including the 'Mother and Child Scheme'. This, coupled with strong electoral support for Noel Browne, made politicians see such a measure as politically expedient. At this stage the mother and child scheme was being developed in the context of a white paper on health services and the respective contributions of voluntary, state and medical personnel. Controversy continued and these matters were not legally resolved until the more controversial aspects of the ensuing Bill were amended: the education of women with respect to motherhood, and compulsory medical examinations of children, were deleted. The Health Bill became law in 1953. As regards medical care it was now free for expectant mothers and infants up to six weeks. Free hospital and specialist care were also offered to children up to the age of six. But the state was not legally empowered to provide information on family planning.

FAMILY PLANNING: LEGISLATIVE CONTROL

Within the church, family planning (including the use of the safe period), was discouraged. Canon McCarthy, writing in the 1940s, argued that the 'indiscriminate diffusion of knowledge of the safe period could easily lead to its indiscriminate use – a situation fraught with calamitous circumstances' (Farmar, 1994, 151). There were exceptions to this Catholic rule, however. If a further pregnancy were life-threatening, a Catholic doctor could explain how the safe period worked and recommend its use. In 1951, Pope Pius XII justified the use of the safe period and in April 1963 the first family planning clinic was opened in Holles Street hospital. It was called a Marriage Guidance Clinic and gave advice on the use of the safe period[3]. By then, many doctors had begun to prescribe the pill as a cycle regulator, but in 1968 the encyclical *Humanae Vitae* reaffirmed the church's opposition to the contraceptive pill.

In 1969 a Fertility Guidance Clinic, supported by the International Planned Parenthood Association, opened in Dublin, and a Family Planning Rights group was formed. While it was illegal to sell contraceptives, the clinic could dispense contraceptives freely, while at the same time requesting 'donations' from its clients. Family planning clinics, despite some local public objections, were subsequently set up in a number of regional towns, prescribing the pill, and dispensing condoms and diaphragms.

This situation might have persisted indefinitely were it not for a Supreme Court case in 1973, *McGee vs. Attorney General*. This case decreed that the right to marital privacy encompassed the right to obtain contraceptives for personal use, so section 17 of the (1935) Act which prohibited the importation of contraceptives was unconstitutional. The Labour Party and Contraception Action Campaign called for a change in the law, but legal change was opposed by the church.

Conflict between both groups continued with no legal change until 1979 when the Minister for Health, Charles Haughey, introduced the Health (Family Planning) Act 1979. He described the Act as 'an Irish solution to an Irish problem'. Contraceptives, including condoms, could be prescribed by GPs for medical reasons, or for *bona fide* family planning purposes. Essentially it was a political compromise: state legislation no longer conformed to Catholic teaching, but the fears of a 'floodgate' had to some extent been heeded. The Contraception Action Campaign (CAP) were unhappy with the restrictive clauses and access to contraception remained a contentious issue. To many, it seemed absurd that one needed a prescription to get condoms.

In 1985 the coalition government amended the legislation, permitting the sale of condoms without prescriptions to those aged 18 or older. The publicity accorded to the AIDS virus, and global safe sex campaigns, facilitated the acceptance of this amendment. While the Catholic church still opposed contraception, Irish people over time adopted fertility control practices. The result has been a considerable reduction in the birth rate, as Table 1 shows. It was not until the 1993 Health (Family Planning) (Amendment) Act that health boards were legally obliged to provide family planning services.

Table 1 gives the birth rate of women aged 15-44, and it shows a gradual increase in the overall birth rate in the sixties and seventies, followed by an accelerated decline in the eighties. This decline can be attributed to a decline in higher order births and the deferment of first pregnancies by younger women.

CHANGING FERTILITY PATTERNS IN IRELAND 1946-1991

TABLE 1 BIRTH RATE BY SELECTED YEARS OF WOMEN AGED 15-44 1947-91

Year	No. of births[*]	No. of women[**]	Birth rate[***]
1946	67,922	626,851	108.35
1951	62,878	591,141	106.35
1961	59,825	502,371	119.08
1971	67,551	545,953	123.70
1981	72,158	760,488	94.80
1991	52,690	776,267	67.80

*Health Statistics 1992, p. 19
**Census 1991 Vol. 2 Table 1C
***No. of births over no. of women × 100.0

Table 2 shows that among women under 25 there was an increase in the birth rate between 1961 and 1971, followed by a decline, which is consistent with the overall pattern in Table 1, but the reduction is greater among the younger cohorts. The birth rate among women aged between 15-24 halved between 1971 and 1991.

TABLE 2 BIRTH RATE FOR WOMEN AGED 15-24 FOR SELECTED YEARS 1961-91

Year	No. of births	No. of women	Proportion single[*]	Birth rate
1961	9,452	212,232	90.5	49.4
1971	18,306	236,244	84.7	77.5
1981	19,338	295,433	83.8	65.4
1991	11,012	293,711	93.7	37.4

*Census 1991 Vol. 2 Table 1C

This may be partly explained by postponed marriages, as the average age at marriage has risen. The third column of Table 2 shows that the proportion of women who were single and aged 15-24 decreased in the seventies and eighties but then increased again in the nineties. In 1925-26, the average age at marriage was 35 for men and 29 for women. By 1977-78, it had declined to 26 for men and 24 for women, but by 1990 it had risen to 28 for men and 26 for women. But the propensity to marry has increased since the sixties. By

1986, 89% of women aged between 35 and 44 were married, as contrasted with 72% in 1951. There is some speculation that marriage rates are now declining among younger cohorts but because of the older age on marriage, this cannot be proven as yet.

While marriage rates *per se* are not controversial, non-marital births are and always have been an issue. The annual report on vital statistics has always given the number of non-marital births, earlier called illegitimate births. In 1947, the statistics simply reported that there were 2,348 illegitimate births equivalent to 3.4 % of total births, as contrasted with 3.8% in Northern Ireland and 5.3% in England and Wales. Since 1953, the report on vital statistics gives a breakdown of births by age and legitimacy/non-marital status and by duration of marriage.

Births to lone parents have been seen as particularly problematic. However, lone parenthood is now a very unclear category so I will focus on teenage mothers to assess changes over time. In 1957, there were 1,033 births to women aged under 20. Only 266 (or 26%) were illegitimate. This contrasts with 2,482 births of which 95% were non-marital in 1995. The actual numbers of births have more than doubled but, more interestingly, the proportion that is non-marital has changed totally over time. Further inspection of the 1957 statistics shows the way in which the actual number of illegitimate births was understated (for present comparative purposes) at that time. The report gives the duration of marriage of these birth mothers. Of the 1,033 legitimate births, 280 (27%) were born to women within 0-8 months of marriage. If we added these nonmarital conceptions we would increase the proportion of illegitimate births to 53%. A further 146 were born to women married between 9-11 months. It must be remembered that social patterns dictated that pregnant women must marry. Hence many so-called illegitimate conceptions were legitimated in what were commonly called 'shot-gun' weddings or marriages that were 'ex necessitate et post crimen'[4].

It is interesting to compare the figures for 1957 with those of 1995. In 1995 there were 2,482 births to women under 20 but the striking difference is that in 1995, only 130 or 5% of these were to married women (i.e. were marital births). So while the number of births to young women has increased, their marital status has changed even more. Marriage patterns have greatly changed, but in addition women are no longer forced or encouraged to 'legitimate' a child via marriage prior to its birth.

Given the decline in the overall birth rate, the proportion of births classified as non-marital has constituted a greater proportion of all births over time, and this has invoked some disquiet. Not too surprisingly, non-marital births tended to be concentrated among women under the age of 25. For instance, in 1995 there were 48,530 births of which 10,788 or 22.2 % were outside marriage.

Closer inspection reveals that the proportion of births outside marriage is negatively associated with age. For instance, in 1995, 95% of all births to women aged under 20 were non-marital births. For women aged 21, 78% of births were outside marriage, for women aged 24, 40% while for women aged 30, the proportion had declined to 9% (Vital Statistics 1995, Table 2, p. 103). Of the latter 6,772 or 62% were to women aged under 25. There is a strong connection between the age at which one gives birth and whether or not it is likely to be a non-marital birth. This connection is exacerbated by an upward trend in the average age of *married* mothers having their first births. Pregnancy and marriage among younger cohorts of Irish women are no longer directly connected as they were in the past. Pregnant women do not have to marry, married women have fewer children and have their first child at a later stage in their married life than previously.

ADOPTION

A second strategy for the management of non-marital conceptions and ensuing non-marital births was adoption. This practice peaked in 1967 when 97% of non-marital births were adopted (McCashin, 1995). Table 3 below shows the numbers of marital births and the proportion adopted for selected years.

TABLE 3 NON-MARITAL BIRTHS AND ADOPTIONS, 1961-1991

Year	Non-marital births	Adoptions	Adoptions as a % of births
1961	975	547	56.1
1971	1,842	1,305	70.8
1981	3,914	1,191	30.4
1991	8,766	590	6.7

Source: derived from McCashin, 1996

This table shows that the proportion of non-marital babies which were subsequently adopted increased from the early sixties. While the numbers adopted remained quite similar at about 1,000 a year, they declined as a proportion of non-marital births. By 1983 only 23% of non-marital babies were adopted and by the 1990s only 7%. Adoptions took place in accordance with the regulations of the Adoption Board established under the Adoption Act of 1952.

ABORTION RATES

While no legislation on the substantive issue has as yet been enacted, Irish woman have travelled to England for abortions. Since the 1967 Abortion Act was passed in Britain, approximately 80,000 Irish women have done so. The number of abortions per 1,000 women aged between 15 and 44 normally resident in the Republic of Ireland was 5.8 in 1994, a slight increase from 5.2 in 1991 (Mahon and Conlon, 1996). This can be contrasted with the higher British rate of 14.8 in 1992. It is quite similar to the rate of 6.0 per 1000 in the Netherlands in 1994 (Mahon and Conlon, 1996). The Netherlands has the lowest abortion rate among countries which have legalised abortion.

While the proportion of non-marital babies being adopted declined, the number of abortions grew. For instance, in 1994 there were 9,450 births outside marriage and 4,590 abortions. We could say that 32% of non-marital conceptions were aborted. 87% of women who had abortions in 1994 were single, which suggests that non-marital pregnancies are still problematic.

This increased incidence of abortion in part accounts for some of the reduction in the birth rate. In 1994, 8.7% of conceptions were aborted. These abortions reduce the incidence of non-marital births, as 79% of women who had abortions in 1994 were single, while the remainder were married, separated, divorced or widowed.

This review of non-marital births shows that over time non-marital conceptions/births have been resolved by marriage, adoption and abortion. These three strategies have each been used by women as strategies to cope with the social stigma and personal consequences of non-marital births. Each in turn is a reflection on the changing nature of the relationship between women and society.

Abortion has been a very controversial and divisive issue in Ireland (Mahon, 1995). Since 1980 there has been a campaign demanding the right to legalised abortion in Ireland. Simultaneously, the Society for the Protection of the Unborn Child (SPUC) campaigned to insert a Constitutional amendment prohibiting abortion. The latter was successful and the amendment was carried in a referendum in 1983. This amendment guarantees explicitly the right to life of the 'unborn' with due regard to the equal right to life of the mother.

ABORTION INFORMATION AND REFERRAL

SPUC proceeded to legally challenge abortion referral and information services, arguing that such services were unconstitutional under Article 40.3.3 of the Constitution. They were successful in their High Court and Supreme Court cases taken against Open Door Counselling and the Well Woman Centre.

However, in 1992, the controversial 'X' case erupted over a fourteen-year-old girl who was raped and whose parents brought her to England to procure an abortion. They inquired from the Gardaí about the procurement of foetal tissue to be used in a court as evidence against her rapist. The gardai sought the advice of the Attorney General and he issued a temporary injunction restraining her from leaving the country. The AG's decision was upheld by the High Court who restrained her from leaving the country for nine months and from procuring an abortion within or without the jurisdiction.

The family then appealed to the Supreme Court, arguing that the girl had suicidal tendencies as a result of her pregnancy and that her life was at risk. The Supreme Court ruled that 'if it is established as a matter of probability that there is a real and substantial risk to the life, as distinct from the health, of the mother, which can only be avoided by the termination of her pregnancy, such termination is permissible, having regard to the true interpretation of Article 40, s 3,sub-s 3 of the Constitution' (Hogan and Whyte, 1994, 799).

According to the Supreme Court, the government would have to introduce appropriate legislation on the issue. However, the court also ruled that only women whose lives were endangered could legally travel to secure an abortion. This was a new restriction. In November of 1992 three new amendments were put to the electorate. The Twelfth Amendment sought to exclude the risk of self-destruction as grounds for abortion and this was rejected by the electorate. The Thirteenth Amendment proposed that Article 40 'shall not limit freedom to travel between the State and another state', while the Fourteenth Amendment related to information and read as follows:

> This subsection shall not limit freedom to obtain or make available, in the State, subject to such conditions as may be laid down by law information relating to services lawfully available in another state.

The Thirteenth and Fourteenth Amendments were both passed by the electorate. Subsequently, the Minister for Health introduced the Regulation of Information (Services Outside State for Termination of Pregnancies) Act, 1995. The Act regulates the dissemination of information on abortion. Such information can only be given if solicited and then as part of non-directive counselling, where options other than abortion are discussed, and where there is no advocacy of abortion: 'It does not permit counselling which promotes abortion or encourages the woman to select it in preference to other options or which amounts to direct abortion referral' (Hogan and Whyte, 1994, 810). This counselling by voluntary agencies and family planning agencies has been assisted financially by the Department of Health. The Act gives due recognition to the right of doctors who are conscientious objectors not to co-operate. There has as yet been no legislation on abortion, *per se*, even though judges in rulings of the Supreme Court have deemed legislation desirable. In 1995 the Department commissioned a study of crisis pregnancies and abortion to see what policies can be introduced to reduce the incidence of unwanted pregnancies and abortions.

Over time, there has been an increasing separation of state policy on reproductive rights from Catholic church policy. This attempt to extend women's reproductive rights was begun in the 1970s by women's groups and organisations. The establishment of a Ministry of State for Women's Affairs and Family Law Reform helped to focus attention on women's needs. The Ministry sought the provision of family planning services. In conjunction with the Department of Health they organised a women's health week which helped to put women's health on the political agenda. The Ministry of Women's Affairs, together with the Irish Cancer Society and Hume Street Hospital, introduced the first cancer screening clinic for women in 1985. The Minister of Women's Affairs' focus on women's health put some pressure on the Department of Health to increase family planning and cancer screening services for women.

DISEASE AND MORBIDITY

A 1994 report revealed that Irish women have the highest incidence of oesophagus, colon, larynx and breast cancer and have the second overall highest incidence of cancer in the EU (Moller-Jensen *et al*, 1990). In 1990, Irish women had a 1 in 11 chance of developing breast cancer and the death rate from cancer has increased since 1970. This remains an unacceptably high level. Early detection is very important for the prognosis of certain kinds of cancer. The Department did not establish a national screening programme until the end of 1996 and many of the appropriate backup facilities including specialists for this service have yet to be established.

On an equally depressing note, the premature mortality rate from ischaemic heart disease is amongst the highest in any of the EU countries and is 70% above the EU average (*Developing a Policy for Women's Health*, 1995, 13). Studies increasingly show a relationship between dietary practices and health. High blood pressure, smoking, obesity and a sedentary life-style can predispose a person to cardiovascular disease. For a country with an advanced and a highly educated population, this is totally unacceptable. Behaviour modification – by far the most effective way of reducing this rate – is the responsibility of Health Promotion. Of course this has long been treated as the

'Cinderella' of the department. But if women's health is to be improved, health promotion is an increasingly important part of the department's remit. A number of recent reports show that there is still much to be accomplished in that area. Smoking, alcohol consumption and a high fat diet all contribute to premature death.

SMOKING AND ALCOHOL CONSUMPTION AMONG IRISH WOMEN

Lung cancer rates among Irish women have been increasing since 1950s. While in 1992 fewer women (29%) than men (38%) smoked, and almost 52% of women as compared with 33% of men never smoked, women who do smoke are less likely to give up smoking. Furthermore, smoking patterns differ by class, with women in higher classes 1-3 more likely to have never smoked (57%) than women in classes 4-6 (47%). Women in higher classes are also more likely to quit smoking. The department recognised in its health discussion document that further research is needed on the reasons why women smoke and continue to smoke in spite of health warnings. I will return later to the class differences noted.

Modernisation has also brought about a change in the consumption of alcohol. A study of drinking patterns showed that older women aged 50-69 were more likely to have never taken alcohol as contrasted with younger women (aged 30-49), only 15% of whom never drank (Irish Heart Foundation, 1994). Class differences were also found, with women in social classes 4-6 more likely (31%) than classes 1-3 (17%) to have never drunk alcohol. Consistent with this, there were more current drinkers in social classes 1-3 (77%) than in social classes 4-6 (60%). However, women are still admitted to psychiatric hospitals for alcoholic disorders though they constitute only 23% of such patients.

DIETARY BEHAVIOUR

A recent Irish review of diet and cancer concluded that there was no evidence to support an association between dietary fat and breast cancer, but high meat intakes were associated with an increased risk of cancer of the colon (*Food Safety Advisory Committee, Diet and Health*, 1994). On balance, that review suggested that the data on diet and cancer were inconsistent. However, they concluded that the evidence linking the antioxidant vitamins and cancer was quite consistent, suggesting that people should increase their consumption of fruit and vegetables. The prevalence of fruit and vegetable consumption was higher among women than men, but overall only 16% consumed more than four portions of fruit and vegetables per day, though 54% of women had between 2 and 3 helpings. Overall 21% of women in classes 1-3 as contrasted with only 12% of women in classes 4-6 had four or more portions (Irish Heart Foundation, 1994, 26). So all women, and especially those in classes 4-6, need to increase their consumption of fruit and vegetables.

PHYSICAL ACTIVITY

More women (32%) than men (25%) were likely to be sedentary during their working day, and they were also more likely to be sedentary than engage in any physical activity in their leisure time (Irish Heart Foundation, 1994, 21). Younger women and women in classes 1-3 were more likely to be active, or very active, but the percentage was small (only 13%). However the study found that more women (62%) than men (44%) were in the 'acceptable' weight category. 10% of both men and women were classified as obese, with slightly more of those coming from classes 4-6. Older women were more prone to obesity.

Overall one can deduce that women are, in general, more likely to live healthy life-styles but that there are class differences visible between them. Middle and upper class women are more receptive to changes in behaviour. In fact it may well be that they more readily adopt a new culture of health. Part of this culture is in keeping with the modern notion of a reflective self – people need to feel that they control their lives to a greater extent. By engaging in healthy behaviour, they will be able to reduce or delay the degenerative processes of the body. The proliferation of health and anti-ageing books is evidence of this. But why are women in some classes more responsive than others to such messages?

Hart (1985, 68-74) argues that smoking may have different values among the working class. One such value is its narcotic effect – a means of reducing the physical stress of work. If this is so it is a material cause rather than a cultural one. If one considers it a pleasurable activity, perhaps one can argue that the middle classes have a greater range of activities and can afford other pleasures, making it easier for them to give up smoking.

She invoked deferred gratification as a more likely explanation. This is a process whereby an activity which would give immediate gratification is deferred or sacrificed in order to get a greater reward much later on. This willingness to defer gratification is more common amongst groups who feel that they have a sense of mastery over their positions in life. Middle-class respondents tend to show greater levels of self-mastery. People in lower socio-economic classes do not exhibit high degrees of self-mastery and have a more fatalistic approach to their lives. Such self-mastery has much to do with one's resources in life, the kind of job one has, money, property and material possessions. Hannan and O'Riain (1993) found that the unemployed feel much less in control of their lives. Breen and Whelan (1996) found that fatalism was related to class, with much higher levels of fatalism among the working class. These feelings of low personal control are seriously damaging to one's well-being. Feelings of control are also reduced by low income, lack of financial or emotional support and social isolation. These concerns cannot be addressed by health promotion alone but depend on eliminating poverty and unemployment.

SEXUAL AND PHYSICAL ABUSE AGAINST WOMEN

One of the aspects of modern society already alluded to is the way in which the private is increasingly subjected to public vigilance. Women have always been victims of rape, sexual assault and domestic violence, but these have only come on the public agenda in recent years. This has in turn created new responsibilities for the Department of Health. In January 1985 Ireland's first sexual assault unit was opened in the Rotunda Hospital, providing specialist investigation and treatment services for adult victims of rape and sexual assault. The work of the rape crisis centres has focused attention on the trauma of rape and sexual abuse and offers counselling and support to victims. The Department of Health contributes to groups offering such services nationally. Such counselling is now seen as very necessary for women, to regain their self-esteem and confidence, thereby avoiding health repercussions later. The Department of Health also contributes to the expenses of running costs of refuges for battered wives and children. But such services are still marginal ones, highly dependent on voluntary effort and unevenly distributed nationally.

THE BLOOD TRANSFUSION SERVICE BOARD AND HEPATITIS C SCANDAL

The years 1994-1997 heralded public exposure of unprofessional practices in the Blood Transfusion Service Board. This was alluded to by a former Assistant Secretary as the greatest health scandal of this century. Women, especially mothers, were the principal victims in the Hep-C scandal. A blood product called Anti-D, which was made by the blood service, was given to women at childbirth to prevent a condition called Rh Haemolytic Disease. This disease affects about 5,000 annually: the problem arises when a mother has Rhesus negative blood but her unborn baby has Rhesus positive blood. After the birth of the first baby, the mother develops anti-bodies to any blood that is left behind. If she were to become pregnant again with a Rhesus positive baby these antibodies would multiply and kill the baby's red blood cells, causing anaemia, brain damage or even death. Anti-D is given to women after birth to prevent this happening, thereby protecting the viability and health of the next foetus.

However, it was discovered that the Anti-D product given to women in 1977 was contaminated with the hepatitis C virus. Hepatitis C (as distinct from hepatitis A and hepatitis B) was not identified until 1989. For those who cannot beat the infection, this virus causes inflammation of the liver and can lead to cirrhosis, cancer of the liver and death. However, the first symptoms are fatigue and general malaise, and women who initially presented with these were not initially diagnosed as having hepatitis C. This only became apparent in 1994, when a large number of female blood donors had signs of hepatitis C. These women had all received anti-D in 1977 (Bowers, 1997). This was subsequently linked with six cases of jaundice which had been reported amongst women who got Anti-D in 1977. Initially it was presumed that the problem was confined to 1977, and women who had received the Anti-D in 1977 were invited to be tested for hepatitis C. However, over time it became apparent that the problem was not confined to one batch of Anti-D. Subsequently all women who had received Anti-D between 1970 and 1994 were invited for testing.

The women affected were all women with young children, for whom the consequences of testing positive for hepatitis C were shattering. They were concerned about themselves and their dependent families. But no admission of responsibility by the BTSB for issuing contaminated Anti-D was initially forthcoming. In fact, the full story might never have emerged without the efforts of Positive Action, a limited company set up by women who were affected by the virus and who live their lives in fear of fatal liver disease.

The full process whereby the hepatitis C scandal was finally fully revealed is itself a study of the intricate difficulties involved in ensuring the public accountability of a national agency. Part of the credit must go to the tenacity and bravery of Brigid McCole. She began a High Court proceeding against the Blood Bank, the Minister for Health, the state and others claiming that she was infected with hepatitis C from contaminated Anti-D. She wished to do so anonymously but that request was refused. An expert group was set up under Dr Miriam Hederman O'Brien to investigate the hepatitis issue in 1994. They reported to the Minister for Health at the end of January and their report was published at the end of April 1995. Its main findings were that Anti-D had become infected from plasma taken from a patient who developed jaundice in late 1976. This infected plasma was used by the Blood Bank to make anti-D. The use of her plasma contravened approved standards for the safe production of Anti-D.

More damning was the finding that the chief medical consultant of the Blood Bank had been informed by Middlesex Hospital in 1991 of a clear link between hepatitis C and Anti-D, and failed to take appropriate action then. The Blood Bank should have withdrawn its Anti-D product and started patient screening at that time. While the report based on evidence supplied by the Blood Bank had not answered all the questions raised, its findings (even if limited) were quite shocking: even after the contaminated Anti-D had been withdrawn in early 1994, it had still been used in nine known cases subsequently. The Blood Bank could not even effectively engage in damage limitation. The Expert Group also identified a second source of infection from the use of a contaminated anti-D donor between 1991 and 1994. They concluded that there had been an absence of internal planning, a medical committee which did not fulfil its functions, and poor management (Bowers, 1997, 70).

Subsequent to the publication of the report a new chief medical consultant and a new chief executive officer were appointed. A tribunal of compensation was also established by the Minister for Health, Michael Noonan. At this juncture others, such as those who had received contaminated product through transfusions, formed Transfusion Positive in April 1995 to represent their interests to the compensation tribunal. The quest for formal compensation was pursued in parallel with the quest for a full disclosure of all the facts of the Blood Bank hepatitis C controversy.

The Bain Consultancy report on the Blood Bank, commissioned by the minister and published in 1995, recommended a complete reorganisation of the Blood Bank, itself an indication that all was not well. The minister resisted the formation of a legal tribunal, but members of Positive Action wanted a statutory tribunal and legal endorsement of the rights to continued medical care. In September 1995, a Tribunal of Compensation was established for all those infected. This would pay compensation on an *ex gratia* basis, but there was no legal admission of responsibility and its proceedings would be in private. This option was offered as an alternative to the High Court proceedings already threatened by many women. Further, if they pursued their cases, their litigation would be defended by the state.

Positive Action was not satisfied. With money secured from the National Lottery, they appointed a co-ordinator to help their campaign. They got legal advice from a former Attorney General and appeared before the Social Affairs Committee. In 1995, an early High Court case hearing was requested by Brigid McCole on grounds of ill health. She wanted confirmation of how she had contracted hepatitis C and of BTSB's liability. Proof of their negligence was being denied to claimants by the Compensation Tribunal. While preparing the case in March 1996, the High Court demanded documents from the Blood

Bank. This included the procurement of a file not made available to the Expert Group. This file, hitherto 'missing', showed that the BTSB knew in 1976-77 that patient X, from whose blood anti-D had been manufactured, had infectious hepatitis. But, the BTSB argued, as Hepatitis C had not been scientifically diagnosed until the eighties they assumed that she had hepatitis B or A. She tested negative for B so they assumed she had A. This was believed not to be passed on through blood, so her plasma – despite these queries – was used again to make anti-D. As this very important file had not been seen by the Expert Group, Positive Action demanded a full judicial inquiry.

Meantime the BTSB were preparing for their High Court case. However, on September 1996, the Blood Bank lawyers wrote to Mrs McCole admitting liability and offering an unreserved apology for her infection. Just before her death, the case was settled between the BTSB and Mrs McCole's legal team. She was awarded £175,000 plus legal costs.

The Minister for Health, under continued pressure, finally agreed to set up a Tribunal of Inquiry into the hepatitis C affair on October 15, 1996. That Tribunal found that the Blood Bank staff had acted unprofessionally and had not followed international best practices in the manufacture of Anti-D. It had not had a licence for fourteen years. To get this licence it was supposed to be inspected by the National Drugs Advisory Board every three years; these inspections had not been carried out. Communication with and supervision of the BTSB by the Department of Health were inadequate. Furthermore, the aftermath of the exposure of the hepatitis C problem was ineffectively handled by the BTSB.

This Tribunal, the exposure of the minutiae of the workings of the BTSB and their admitted liability, must surely have altered any public servant's sense of public accountability. The tireless action of the Positive Action group won out in the end. The entire truth was revealed and a statutory Compensation Tribunal was established. However, the Tribunal had revealed that appointed boards were not sufficiently vigilant or impartial to oversee the activities of their employees. Formal procedures were neglected over time, and the Department of Health and the National Drugs Advisory Board had not been sufficiently vigilant. Finally, and perhaps surprisingly to many who expect high standards from professional medical staff, the unprofessional activities of the Blood Bank staff and the continuity of such conduct over time showed that they needed supervision.

But the scandal also showed a new relationship between the Department of Health and the public. No longer was the church or any medical association centre stage; instead one saw an example of 'people power' in action. Positive Action, set up initially as a support group, became a force to be reckoned with. While the enormity of the scandal no doubt helped the group to mobilise opinion, the activities of the department are likely in the future to be increasingly subjected to such public scrutiny.

The respective responsibilities of the department and its many professional staff will need to be firmly delineated. The responsibility of members appointed to boards needs to be clearly outlined, and they must be made aware that they are accountable for the organisation's practices. Effective procedures for ensuring best practices need to be established. All patients are now customers with rights and expect quality care. Patients will increasingly resort to litigation if they are dissatisfied. Sadly, the women in Positive Action had to fight to win their case, but their action will have helped to alter the nature of the relationship between the department and its public.

A WOMAN-FRIENDLY HEALTH POLICY

While Positive Action showed that women could be empowered, women are still under-represented in positions of responsibility in the health services. In 1995, only 13% of members of health boards were women. On other boards under the aegis of the department only 32% were women. Women are also under-represented at consultant level – in 1990 only 16% of 1,025 practising consultants were female. This under-representation is particularly acute in obstetric and gynaecological areas, where only 3% of consultants are women. Only three of the most senior posts at management level were occupied by women in 1995. There has been no female secretary of the Department of Health, though a woman has recently been appointed as assistant secretary. Women do, however, represent an increasing proportion of those in middle management which must augur well for the future. However, a study in the Mid-Western Health Board revealed that male organisational culture represented an obstacle to the promotion of women (O'Connor, 1996). A newly-established Office for Health Management has been set up to develop management and this includes creating more opportunities for its female staff. On-going monitoring of gender equity will be required to ensure organisational change.

The Commission on the Status of Women in its 1993 report noted that women should have greater input into the formulation of health policy. The department responded positively to that proposal and as a result of consultations published *Developing a Policy for Women's Health*. This examined the health services from a woman's point of view and identified the priorities for improvement. This in turn led to the formulation and adoption of a health policy for women in 1997. The policy identified the following priorities: a reduction in smoking; screening of breast and cervical cancer and their effective treatment; woman-friendly maternity services; services for victims of domestic violence and rape; and a programme for the special needs of traveller women. But such policies must be actively pursued and significant gains made in these areas, otherwise such policy documents are at best exercises in public relations.

That review was a significant and welcomed departure in that it actively consulted women's groups in addition to health boards, medical representatives and social partners. Such consultations have in turn raised expectations and no doubt the implementation of those policies will be eagerly monitored. Women themselves have finally, fifty years after the formation of the department, been given a voice and some input into the formation of health policy. No doubt pressure groups and consumer groups will increasingly demand more and better services. A more informed and educated public will make greater demands on the health service. Its published plans have already created a sense of entitlement that will extend the nature and range of its services. The next fifty years will undoubtedly see the further empowerment of women and further attendant improvements in their life expectancy and in the quality of their lives.

REFERENCES

1.   This is to be contrasted with men's life expectancy of 64.5 in 1950-52 and 72.3 in 1990-92.

2.   The 1947 statistics refer to these as deaths caused by or associated with pregnancy, childbirth and the puerperal state.

3.   It was opened with the tacit support of Achbishop McQuaid, though Arthur Barry and Eamon de Valera, two prominent Dublin obstetricians, walked out of the proposal meeting and a number of nurses resisted involvement. (See Farmar 1994).

4.   F. Kelly notes that this was the reason for some marriages of brides under 20 (See p. 27, *Window on a Catholic Parish. Maynooth Studies in Local History*, Irish Academic Press 1966).

CHAPTER 8

Out of the Shadow – Developing Services for the Elderly

Davis Coakley

Most people in Ireland today can expect to live into old age. This is in striking contrast to the situation at the beginning of the century when life expectancy was around fifty years. This dramatic change has come about largely due to changes in living standards and to a lesser extent in health care. It has been one of the great triumphs of modern civilisation. However, the new demographic structure also presents us with certain challenges and one of these is ensuring the provision of appropriate facilities to cope with the increasing number of sick and disabled elderly people in our society. Ireland has been slow to meet this challenge and our responses have been heavily conditioned by historical factors. In this chapter I describe the historical framework in which our current services developed, I then outline the attempts which have been made in the last thirty years to escape from this history and I conclude by highlighting some of the areas which I believe need urgent attention now.

OLD AGE IN CELTIC IRELAND

In Celtic society, as in many other ancient traditions, old age was apparently greatly honoured. The so-called Brehon Laws contain several enlightened provisions for the maintenance of old people who were no longer able to support themselves. When the head of a family became too old to manage his affairs he could hand over his land to his son on the understanding that he would be supported for the rest of his life. If he did not choose to live with his son a separate house was to be constructed for him, the dimensions of which were described in detail in the law. Owners of land who did not have children could sign over their property to a third party on a similar understanding of continued maintenance. Older people with means were able to negotiate lodging in a local monastery when they were no longer able to support themselves (Joyce, 1906).

According to late transcriptions of the 'Brehon Laws', there were strict regulations regarding the support of older individuals without means. This duty usually fell to the children or foster children and the clan became responsible for destitute older people without children. Arrangements included boarding out and an early form of outdoor relief. There was also the equivalent of a welfare officer in ancient Irish society. He was called *'Uaithne'* and his task was to ensure that the poor were supported. He received an allowance for this duty and it was anticipated because of the nature of his task that he would receive considerable abuse from time to time. A special provision was made within the law that he could bear these attacks on his honour without his family or himself being under any obligation to respond to them!

In medieval Ireland the monasteries played an important role in caring for older people who required shelter and care. The suppression of the monasteries and the defeat of the Irish clan system in the sixteenth and seventeenth centuries brought about the collapse of these ancient systems of support for the elderly and the poor. The dramatic change in land ownership meant that new support systems could not emerge from the ruins of the old Celtic world. As a result there was widespread misery and suffering throughout the country in the seventeenth and eighteenth centuries. A number of individuals were moved to take action and this period saw the emergence of the voluntary hospital system in Dublin with the foundation of Dr Steevens's Hospital, Mercer's Hospital and the Meath Hospital.

POOR LAW SYSTEM

The development of the poor law system in England during the eighteenth century identified the support of the aged and the poor as a parochial responsibility. Parish overseers were given the power to raise money so that resources became available to support the elderly and the poor in the local community. However, the poor law system did not apply in Ireland and as a result a community-based system of supporting the poor did not evolve. When the authorities did begin to make provision for the relief of the poor and destitute in Ireland at the beginning of the eighteenth century, the response was largely an institutional one. The first workhouse in Ireland was erected in 1703 on a site now occupied by St James's Hospital in Dublin. Designed primarily to cope with beggars, disorderly women and orphans, it soon had to house an increasing number of disabled elderly people.

In 1832 a royal commission was established by the British government to enquire into the practical application of the laws for the relief of the poor in England and Wales. The commission was primarily concerned with the provisions for the able-bodied poor and it recommended that there should be a move from outdoor relief to an institutional approach. It was decided that the able-bodied person would receive relief only in a workhouse where the conditions were to be less tolerable than those of the poorest labourers in the community. In 1838 the government sent George Nicholls, one of the English poor law commissioners, to Ireland with the task of introducing the workhouse system. The country was divided into unions and within a very short period 130 workhouses were opened. Although designed originally to house unemployed able-bodied men and women under spartan conditions, the workhouses gradually began to change function and were increasingly used as institutions to house the elderly and infirm. The inmates of the workhouses lived under appalling conditions and there were constant demands for reform throughout the nineteenth century, particularly when the system almost collapsed during the Great Famine. A Vice-Regal Commission on Poor Law Reform recommended in 1906 that the aged and infirm should be moved from the workhouses to institutes to be known as county alms-houses, but this recommendation was not implemented.

THE INTRODUCTION OF COUNTY HOMES

In the general election of December 1918 Sinn Féin was given an overwhelming mandate to set up an independent Irish parliament in Dublin. The first Dáil Éireann adopted a programme which included an aspiration to introduce more humane facilities for the elderly, declaring that the aged and infirm 'shall no longer be regarded as a burden but rather entitled to the nation's gratitude and consideration' (O'Connor, 1995). Between 1921 and 1922 the Minister for Local Government began to dismantle the poor law system. County councils were given responsibility for the relief of the poor. Most of the workhouses were closed but thirty-three were maintained as county homes. It was envisaged that these county homes would provide care for the aged and infirm. However, in effect the county homes continued to provide care for several different categories such as unmarried mothers, orphaned children and the mentally retarded. A government report in 1927 identified the essentials for a county home as 'good water supply and sanitary and bathing accommodation, well ventilated walls, good diets, sufficient dormitory accommodation, good kitchen and laundry arrangements and possibly, above all, a sympathetic and maternal administration' (Relief

Commission, 1927). The recommendations were in marked contrast to reality, as several of the homes had no water supply and no bathing or sanitary accommodation. Many of the elderly people admitted to county homes deteriorated rapidly as there was no provision of occupational or diversional therapy.

The Irish government established an inter-departmental committee in 1949 consisting of representatives from the Departments of Health, Finance, Social Welfare and Local Government to examine the question of the reconstruction and replacement of the county homes. The committee found that there were approximately 8,500 inmates in county homes at that time and approximately 5,000 of these were over the age of 55. A significant number of unmarried mothers, orphans, mentally retarded children and adults were still housed in the county homes. The findings of the committee were uninspiring and they reiterated the main recommendations of the 1927 committee. The county homes were to be retained but they should admit only the aged and the chronic sick. Specialised accommodation was to be provided for the other categories. The committee, although aware of the trend in other countries towards smaller homes for the elderly needing care, recommended the retention of large institutions. They actually found attractions in the design of the old workhouses for this purpose.

A LANDMARK REPORT

By the end of the 1960s there was an increasing awareness of the growing numbers of people aged 65 years and over in society. There was also a greater public appreciation of the right of the elderly to share in the rising living standards in the country.

A number of schemes were introduced by the Department of Social Welfare which did enhance the quality of life of older people. These schemes included free travel facilities, free electricity allowance and free radio and television. In 1968 an inter-departmental government committee chaired by J. J. Darby reported on the care of the aged in Ireland. This committee concluded that services for the elderly which until then had been almost entirely confined to the destitute should begin to embrace other classes in Irish society. In line with previous reports the committee decried the general standard of institutional accommodation and demanded that it should be raised progressively. However, this committee differed from its predecessors in that it placed great emphasis on the importance of maintaining the older person as long as possible in the community. The committee considered that the aims of services provided for the elderly should be:

(*a*) to enable the aged who can do so to continue to live in their own homes;

(*b*) to enable the aged who cannot live in their own homes to live in other similar accommodation;

(*c*) to provide substitutes for normal homes for those who cannot be dealt with as at (*a*) or (*b*) and

(*d*) to provide hospital services for those who cannot be dealt with as at (*a*), (*b*), or (*c*).

The report stressed the importance of developing community services for the elderly. It advocated improvements in a range of medical and nursing services in the community. It recommended that occupational therapy, social workers and chiropody should be made available on a community basis and that physiotherapy should be available in all community areas on an out-patient basis. The committee also suggested that health authorities should introduce 'boarding out' schemes as a normal feature of their services for the elderly. The practice of 'boarding out', with private householders, elderly people who could no longer live alone was being introduced in a number of European countries. It was thought that a boarding out scheme could be very successful in Ireland provided that careful selection of the persons being boarded out and of the persons to receive them was made.

The committee advocated radical reform in institutional care of the elderly. They criticised the fact that elderly people were being admitted to county homes without any medical or social assessment and without any effort to determine whether some form of community intervention would have obviated the need for admission. The report advocated the establishment of geriatric assessment units within the general hospital. It was envisaged that patients would be admitted for short periods of treatment and rehabilitation and that they would then be discharged home or assigned to the most appropriate accommodation. The report also supported the development of day hospitals where patients could receive treatment during the day and return to their own homes at night. Day hospitals were to have a defined medical function and were not to be seen as social support.

The committee recommended the development of welfare homes for frail elderly people who could no longer cope at home but who did not need intensive nursing care. These homes would provide as far as possible the atmosphere of a normal home and it was suggested that each home should have not more than thirty or forty places. The committee also proposed the establishment of a National Council for the Aged whose purpose would be to promote in every way possible the general welfare of the elderly and to co-ordinate the efforts of voluntary and public services at national level.

MORE ENLIGHTENED POLICIES

Government policy towards the elderly was heavily influenced by the 1968 report. Steps were taken to bring about a real increase in the value of the old age pension. The contributory pension for an eligible couple almost doubled in real terms between 1966 and 1985 and the non-contributory pension increased by 60%. Many other benefits for the elderly were either introduced or increased. The qualifying age for pensions was reduced from seventy to sixty-six and the means testing was eased. A free telephone rental system for social welfare pensioners aged sixty-six and over was also introduced.

Approximately thirty welfare homes were constructed in different parts of the country. There were also substantial improvements in housing for the elderly. From the early 1970s local authorities allocated about 10% of local authority dwellings to the elderly and disabled and sheltered housing schemes were established. Specialist schemes were introduced to carry out repairs in the homes of elderly people owning their own homes. However, despite the general improvement in housing for the elderly, certain sections of the elderly population remained considerably disadvantaged. This was particularly true of elderly single person households. A report on incomes of the elderly in 1984 which was carried out by the National Council for the Aged found that 12% of the elderly who depended mainly on income from social welfare pensions and 18% of the elderly living alone were existing in conditions which were defined as 'absolute' poverty.

In 1972 the dispensary medical service was replaced by the general medical service and this gave eligible persons a choice of general practitioner, resulting in greater home visiting by doctors to the elderly. Considerable developments took place in the domiciliary nursing services provided in all parts of the country. At-risk registers were introduced by public health nurses and services such as home-help, meals on wheels and day care services for the elderly were developed by both voluntary bodies and health boards. A drugs users' scheme was introduced in 1971 which benefited elderly persons without medical cards and allowed them to recoup the cost of drugs. The appointments of directors of community care teams and medical officers of health within the health boards provided a new framework for the development of services for the elderly. Eligibility for treatment in public hospitals was extended to the entire population in 1979. There was considerable development also within the voluntary sector. Almost all meals-on-wheels and laundry services, and about half of the home-help services, together with a significant proportion of the day care services for the elderly, were being run by voluntary organisations in the 1970s. The establishment of the National Social Service Council in 1973 provided support for these voluntary bodies. Training and advisory programmes were established and community information services were developed as a result.

GERIATRIC MEDICINE

Comhairle na nOispidéal, the body responsible for approving the creation of consultant posts, recommended in 1975 that geriatric departments should be staffed by properly trained whole-time specialists in geriatric medicine. Since then the Comhairle has supported the development of geriatric medicine as a speciality, a commitment reiterated in a further report published in 1985. In more recent years the Comhairle has also supported the appointment of specialists in old age psychiatry. The publication in 1991 of the Dublin Hospital Initiative Report on acute hospitals gave further impetus to the development of geriatric medicine. The report emphasised that the acute care of older patients was a core responsibility of the acute hospitals and that these hospitals should have the appropriate facilities and organisational policies in place to cope with this aspect of their workload.

OLD AGE PSYCHIATRY

Studies have shown that the majority of elderly people suffering from mental illness remain undetected and untreated in the community. It has been estimated that only 10% of people with a mental illness are in contact with services. There is a great need for epidemiological studies in this area, and a national strategy for services for people with mental illness and their carers is an urgent necessity. The comprehensive treatment of mental disorders in older people must involve co-ordinated action by local government, social services, health services, the voluntary sector and specialist services (National Council for the Aged, 1988).

The development of old age psychiatry as a speciality must now receive the kind of attention which has been given to the development of geriatric medicine over the last decade. At present there are only four old age psychiatrists in the country, whereas it has been estimated that approximately thirty old age psychiatrists are needed to provide an adequate service throughout the country.

THE NATIONAL COUNCIL FOR THE AGED

The National Council on Ageing and Older People was originally established in 1981 as the National Council for the Aged. The council advises the Minister for Health on all aspects of ageing and the welfare of older people either on its own initiative or at the request of the Minister. Since its inception, the council has based its advice on systematic research on a wide range of topics relevant to the welfare of older people in Ireland and to their carers. This research has been published in a series of nearly fifty publications on a diverse range of issues. These include publications on housing, income maintenance, institutional care, transport and access to services, day centres, carers in the home, nursing home and dementia. The Council has also looked at the quality of life of older Irish people in different settings. The Council has been particularly active in addressing the problems of negative attitudes to ageing and older people. This has been a central theme of many of its publications. The Council was instrumental in the inception of *Age and Opportunity*, an independent voluntary organisation dedicated to challenging negative attitudes to ageing and encouraging greater participation by older people in all aspects of Irish society.

THE YEARS AHEAD

Although much had been achieved within two decades of publication of the Care of the Aged report, there were still many major challenges to be faced. In 1986 the Minister for Health established a working party under the chairmanship of Dr Joseph Robins. This working party concluded that although many improvements had taken place there were still significant gaps, particularly in areas relating to the most vulnerable elderly. The Report of the Working Party, *The Years Ahead . . . A Policy for the Elderly*, was published in 1988. It was a comprehensive report which made over a hundred main recommendations.

The Years Ahead placed great emphasis on the importance of focusing as much care as possible on the elderly in their own homes. Recommendations were made in relation to public health and liaison nursing, family practitioners, and domiciliary services embracing occupational therapy, physiotherapy, speech therapy and chiropody. The report recommended that the main emphasis in housing policy for the elderly should be to enable elderly people to choose between adapting their own homes to the increasing disabilities of old age or to move to accommodation more suited to their needs. Priority should be given to improving the accommodation of elderly people lacking basic amenities. This was a sensible approach given that 80% of elderly householders were owner occupiers. The report stressed the importance of good liaison between statutory and voluntary bodies. It was recommended that where it was not feasible to maintain elderly persons in their own homes or in ordinary local authority houses, sheltered housing should be considered as the first alternative.

The Years Ahead has had considerable influence on the development of services for the elderly in recent years. Care teams focusing on the needs of the elderly in the community have been introduced, and co-ordinators of services for the elderly have been appointed in community care areas. Community hospitals have also been developed and they have made valuable contributions to respite and day care. Liaison between statutory and voluntary bodies has improved but there remains a need for much greater co-operation. This is particularly true in relation to housing needs where an integrated plan which would enhance all sectors is badly needed. Major deficiencies still exist, particularly in the range of domiciliary services available. Where services have been developed at centralised locations in the community, access to them is often difficult because of the lack of adequate transport arrangements. Some health boards have been far less assiduous than others in introducing the recommendations of *The Years Ahead*. One of the major reasons for this was the failure to put a legislative framework in place which would have given the recommendations a statutory status.

TEACHING AND RESEARCH

There is a great need for educational programmes on ageing and the elderly for all professions involved in health care. Although some teaching in this area appears on the curriculum of most professional schools it is still very inadequate. The Department of Health and the Higher Education Authority should become much more proactive in this area. Caring for elderly patients is a major part of the task of most health care professionals and they should be introduced to the subject in their undergraduate years. There is also a great need for academic development in this area for postgraduate students. One of the encouraging recent developments has been the introduction of an MSc Course in Gerontological Nursing at Trinity College. Academic development in geriatric medicine has been very slow in Ireland. At present there is only one chair in the discipline and this is based at Trinity College, in marked contrast to the situation in the United Kingdom where virtually all the medical schools have full departments of geriatric medicine.

There has been a growing interest in research into the care of the elderly as reflected in the increasing number of high quality presentations at meetings of the Irish Gerontological Society. The society has the particular advantage of being multi-disciplinary and this is reflected in the wide range of topics discussed. The National Council on Ageing and Older People has produced an impressive body of work in collaboration with a number of third level institutions over the years. The Mercer's Institute for Research on Ageing (MIRA) was established in 1987 at St James's Hospital with funding from the assets of Mercer's Hospital. The work of the institute has concentrated primarily on Alzheimer's disease and on respiratory infections in the elderly. It has established the first memory clinic in the country for patients with Alzheimer's disease and related illnesses. Recently the Department of Health has decided to establish a Dementia Information and Development Centre which will also be based at St James's Hospital. This new centre will liaise with similar centres in other countries. Its main purpose will be to provide information education and training for private, statutory and voluntary service providers working with dementia sufferers and their carers.

PROMOTING HEALTH IN OLD AGE

Good health in old age is obviously a great advantage for the individual but it also has important implications for the state. The more elderly people who enjoy an active old age the less demand there will be on government resources. The incidence of many diseases rises with age and the mortality associated with these diseases also increases. This places increased demands on the acute services and also on support services both in the hospital and in the community. There is surprisingly little information available on the health status of our elderly population, and less on how it changes over time. Heart disease, stroke, malignancy and respiratory disease are the major causes of mortality in the older age group. The major causes of morbidity are cerebrovascular and cardiovascular disease, impaired vision and hearing, osteoporosis and osteoarthritis, incontinence, dementia and depression. Considerable attention is being focused on attempts to reduce the total period of disability at the end of life and there is increasing emphasis as a result on improving the quality of life of older people.

There is an unwarranted pessimism surrounding the whole area of preventative medicine in old age. This is in part due to the absence of properly constructed treatment trials in this age group. Old people are usually excluded from trials. Yet in the exceptional incidences where elderly people have been included in well constructed major trials, the results often reveal benefit for that group. For instance it has been shown that the control of hypertension in the elderly can reduce the risk of coronary heart disease and stroke, that older patients benefit from thrombolytic therapy and that the treatment of depression and anxiety produces results as good as those achieved in younger people. Indeed it has been shown in some trials that the benefits of treatment can sometimes be greater in the older age groups. Considerably more attention should be given in future years to the whole role of preventative medicine in ageing. If successful strategies are to be adopted they must be based on sound evidence. This again emphasises the importance of properly constructed research. Education both of the public and health care professions is also critical in this area.

TREATING ILLNESS

There is a widespread belief in society that older people benefit less from medical and surgical interventions than do people of younger age. It is a view shared by some health care professionals who use age as a criterion for the exclusion of old people from certain forms of health care. Some doctors have a higher threshold for referral of older patients to certain specialist services. Actions and attitudes such as these cannot be substantiated by research. In fact there is a considerable body of evidence accumulating which would suggest that older people benefit considerably from the advances which have been made in both medicine and surgery over the last few decades. For example it has been shown that in intensive care, provided sufficient information is available about an individual's physiological status, the age of the patient contributes very little extra to the prediction of outcome. Older people are a heterogeneous group so there can be no justification for the use of chronological age as a proxy for biological fitness when making decisions on the investigation and treatment of illness in old age.

Approaches to the provision of health care for the elderly can be broadly divided into two categories – the therapeutic approach and the prosthetic approach. The therapeutic approach seeks to investigate and treat any illnesses which may be impairing the performance of an older person, and it places stress on the importance of rehabilitation. The emphasis is on the preservation of the patient's autonomy and independence. In contrast, prosthetic care seeks to compensate for disability by the provision of a range of supporting services. Prosthetic care is indicated when therapeutic interventions are not appropriate or when they have failed to produce the results required. As a general principle, the prosthetic approach should only be adopted when it is not possible to improve the performance of an individual through therapeutic options.

CARER SUPPORT

Although there have been many changes in Irish society over the last twenty years the family still occupies a central position in caring; the majority of the disabled elderly continue to be cared for at home rather than in institutions. It is only in recent years that the contribution of carers has been recognised by health care policy makers in this country. Some carers become highly stressed and may be receiving little support from local health services or from other family members. Many of those involved in caring give up employment and virtually all forego the possibility of ensuring their own financial independence. They may also be compromising financial arrangements which would give them security in their old age. It is vital that this area should receive much more attention. There is a need to develop further a whole range of support services for carers which should include respite care, home help services, day care services, allowances, information, training and counselling.

ADVANCES IN COMMUNICATION TECHNOLOGY

The advances in computer and communication technology which are currently taking place will have a major impact on the lives of the elderly in the next century. Programmes are already in place in a number of European countries which link the elderly in their homes to a whole range of services in the community. Apart from giving direct access to services such as banking and shopping, technology is being used increasingly to link disabled elderly and their carers with community and hospital services and their family doctors. There is considerable support at European level for developments of this nature.

VIOLENCE AND THE ELDERLY

One of the most disturbing features of life in Ireland in recent years has been the increasing level of violence. There have been many vicious attacks against elderly people living in their own homes, particularly in isolated areas. These have received considerable publicity. However, it has been shown that the health of older people can be significantly affected by what might be described as minor violence and harassment. Many elderly people subjected to abuse of this nature can become seriously ill and some of them opt for institutional care. As a result we have a rather bizarre situation where the victims rather than the perpetrators of the crimes end up in institutional care. Many older people live in fear and some are subjected to repeated attacks. Excuses are made too readily for those who target vulnerable elderly people like this. One can accept that there are many issues involved and solutions are not always easy; however, as a problem it needs concentrated government attention so that necessary steps are taken to deal with it. It should be totally unacceptable to us as a society that the last years of the lives of so many people in this country can be blighted by the experience or fear of violence.

FACILITIES FOR LONG-TERM CARE

Even with ready access to good treatment facilities it is inevitable that some patients with major disabilities will need long-term institutional care. The number of patients needing care of this nature will continue to increase over the next decade because of demographic changes. It has been estimated that there will be over half a million people over the age of sixty-five in Ireland by the year 2011. Contrary to commonly-held perceptions, economic projections predict that we will have the necessary funding to provide adequate services and facilities (ESRI, 1997). Factors such as declining unemployment, increased productivity and an expanding workforce mean that the country will be in a much stronger position to support those members in society who need assistance than it was a decade ago. The scare stories which appear in the media from time to time about the future burden of pensions on the state are not justified. The reality is that in this country overall dependency levels are dropping. It has been estimated that by the year 2020 there will be about a million more people aged 15-64 in the country. There were 230 dependants for every 100 at work in the mid 1980s, whereas it has been predicted that by the year 2010 this will have fallen to 125 per 100. This dividend presents policy makers with a great opportunity to develop a proper modern infrastructure to care for the elderly.

It is essential therefore that appropriate plans are put in place as soon as possible. A sensible and well planned investment spread over a number of years will avoid major problems in the future. We cannot plead ignorance as we have all the figures necessary to justify immediate developments. It cannot be acceptable to go on using older buildings which we have found unsuitable for other purposes to house elderly patients needing specialised care and facilities. Neither is it acceptable that the health boards should become too dependent on the private nursing home sector, which has seen a rapid expansion in recent years. More choice must be introduced into the system and more emphasis must be placed on the quality of the services provided both in the community and in institutions. Private nursing homes are currently inspected under the Health Act (1990) and this helps to ensure standards. However, provision should also be made for the inspection of facilities run by health boards and other agencies involved in the care of older people.

CONCLUSION

Opportunities must be created in our society which will allow older people to lead meaningful and rewarding lives. If this does not occur the burden of ill health and dependency will increase as it does in all marginalised communities. Policies of inclusiveness must be developed in all aspects of life and a major effort must be made to remove the stereotypes which are currently so prevalent.

Health services for the elderly have improved over the last thirty years but much remains to be achieved. It has taken us a long time to move out of the shadow of the workhouse. Now we should be able to plan with more imagination and confidence for the future. We must develop an infrastructure which will support the frail elderly at home and which will also provide them with high quality institutional care when it is needed. We must move to a situation where the elderly are offered choices rather than ultimatums. As a step in this direction, older people should be consulted when planning new services. There is a window of opportunity now to get things right for the elderly in this country. It is essential that the government and its policy makers will have the commitment and vision to make it happen.

CHAPTER 9

People with Disabilities and the Health Services

Anne Colgan

INTRODUCTION

The extraordinary growth and development in the volume, distribution, cost and structure of services available to people with disabilities in Ireland over the past fifty years is one of the most immediately obvious features of this half century. Less obvious, but equally influential, are the shifts in thinking, in ideology, in attitudes, in spheres of influence and in expectations whose evolution has underpinned the services and their delivery structures.

How might those changes be seen to impact on the life of a child born with a disability today, compared with her counterpart of fifty years ago? Today's child with cerebral palsy or other physical disability would in all likelihood spend their childhood in their family surroundings, and have a reasonable expectation that they would attend the local school. Extensive surgical intervention aimed at removing or reducing the physical 'defect' would not be the norm. Local physiotherapy services, though possibly more difficult to access regularly than the family might wish, would be available. Depending on personal capacities, third level education would be a reasonable and attainable goal; technological and mechanical aids could greatly enhance independence.

This child of the late 1990s can look forward to having the choice of living at home, with the support of a personal assistant; the problems of physical access within the home are a removable barrier to living with the family. Travel abroad is possible and usual. This child's expectations about the future and the expectations of others for her would probably be positive and high. Similar experiences would await a child with a learning disability. While any reader with a disability would undoubtedly point to gaps, rigidities, waiting lists and a host of barriers also facing this child, the fact of the times are that changed attitudes, changed professional practices, increases in resource allocation, technical developments and political resolve have all conspired positively over the past fifty years to make possible a high quality of life, in today's terms, for the disabled child of today's generation, even if a whole range of restrictions and barriers often block the path to availing of today's possibilities.

The experience of the child of the late 1940s would probably have been very different. The norm of institutionalisation would have meant an early move away from family and friends, probably for life. For those staying at home, the family attitude of Shame and fear might well have meant a life of isolation more impoverished and isolated than that experienced in an institution. Active and regular surgical intervention in the case of children with physical 'defects' would not have been unusual. Paddy Doyle, in his account of a childhood spent in institutional care, describes in harrowing detail the repeated experimental brain surgery through which doctors tried to address his rare physical condition (Doyle, 1989). In her in-depth account of the life experience of thirty people with physical disabilities, *Pegged Down*, Jean Tubridy points to the common practice of active surgical intervention in the case of babies and children with cerebral palsy. Extensive hospitalisation shaped the lives of children, while doctors looked for cures for little understood disabilities. Minimal services were available and these were centralised in orthopaedic hospitals. Only the most committed parents would be able to make the regular trips to attend hospital clinics, without the benefit of travel passes or domiciliary care allowances to help with costs of travel, and facing inhospitable environments which were still a long way from being the subject of public investment or awareness about access.

The expectations for children with disabilities were often very low. One participant in Jean Tubridy's study tells how, following an assessment, his mother was told 'he has quite a high intelligence, but one would question the advisability of spending a lot of money on education for him'. This did not happen in 1947, but in the mid 1960s, a pointer to the accelerated pace of change in attitude in recent years. Those who succeeded in overcoming the barriers inherent in the society of the day, and in making use of their talents and abilities, often did so on account of the energy, passion and dogged determination of their mothers. One might argue that Christy Browne's story would not happen today, but then one thinks of author Christopher Nolan and poet Davoren Hanna, and their mothers. Personal achievements above the odds and against the odds will be a feature of any age.

INFLUENCES ON CHANGE

The changes experienced by today's young person with a disability have been the outcome of a confluence of several strands of development and influence.

Legislation, economic development, medical and technological advances, advances in thinking about service delivery methods, political and cultural influences have all contributed to shaping the present landscape of services and models of service delivery. To this list of influences we must add the impact of our public servants' inclination to look to developments in Britain in the early years of the independent state, and to model these developments in Ireland. In more recent years, the impact of American and European thinking has, in very different ways, helped to shape and contour our responses to disability.

The setting up of the Department of Health and the passing of the 1947 Health Act laid the foundation for today's health services. In the circumstances of the day, where the focus of public policy was on the control of disease and the development of basic health services, it is not surprising that legislative provision for support and welfare services for people with disabilities was not the focus of this legislation, and had to await much later development.

Ruth Barrington's account of the tensions during that period between government, on the one hand, and the Catholic church and the medical profession on the other, highlights in a dramatic way the sources of power and influence in the Ireland of the day (Barrington, 1987). From the perspective of people with disabilities, perhaps the most significant aspect of service and legislative developments was the manner in which the ethos of the 1937 Constitution, with its strong embodiment of Catholic social teaching, reinforced the role of the voluntary sector in the provision of services to people with disabilities in Ireland. The minimalist role envisaged for the state, and the strong presence of the religious bodies in the field of mental handicap in particular, created a service structure which has retained its general shape and format to the present day. This structure has had lasting consequences for patterns of investment in services, and in the varying pace of development of services for particular groups of disabled people. The role of the voluntary sector in service provision and in innovation has been truly remarkable. However, the state/voluntary division of responsibility has arguably resulted in a pattern of service development which has reflected the zeal of individuals or groups with the vision and energy to initiate services for particular groups, rather than a systematic national response to the needs of all people with disabilities.

CULTURE OF INDEPENDENCE

The introduction of the Disabled Person's Maintenance Allowance in the 1953 Health Act was a significant development for people with disabilities. It represented a move away from poor law provisions and laid the foundations of the system of income maintenance for people with disabilities which has endured to the present day – a very basic requirement for independence and self-determination. However, the location of this allowance within the Department of Health may have created a psychological climate of low expectations among recipients that they could ever work or attempt training for employment. The fears of losing the allowance and its attendant benefits inevitably deterred people from risk-taking around employment opportunities.

Of course, these kinds of rigidities have applied throughout the social welfare system. They were a product of their time and have been gradually modified as insight and understanding of their impact has grown. The DPMA is now in process of being transferred to the Department of Social Welfare. This move, together with the implementation of income support proposals contained in the Report of the Commission on the Status of People with Disabilities in 1996, should the government adopt these, will undoubtedly lend itself to a more flexible, accessible system of income support which will facilitate a stronger culture of independence rather than supporting a culture of dependence. Unfortunately, the problem of the establishment of a training allowance for people with disabilities attending special training centres, equivalent to the FAS allowance, is still unresolved. Recommendations aimed at introducing a training allowance were first mooted in the Green Paper, *Towards a Full Life,* in 1984, and again in the Report of the Commission on the Status of People with Disabilities in 1996. This is one of a small number of issues and practices which have proven to be almost intractable, in spite of general recognition of the need for change, over a twenty-year period. Other examples of issues which impact on significant numbers of people with disabilities, and which appear to have a stubborn resistance to being addressed, include the administrative issue of data on the needs of people with disability for planning purposes, and the position, status and pay of people in sheltered work situations.

LEGAL AND ADMINISTRATIVE STRUCTURES

When we look at the impact of legislation on the lives of people with disabilities over the past fifty years, the 1970 Health Act is most significant. The structural changes introduced by the Act in setting up the health board system finally separated the delivery of health services from the work of the local authorities. This development can be seen as an important step in the devolution of power from the centre to the periphery and as an appropriate separation of the policy function from the policy execution function. On the other hand it could be viewed, retrospectively, as an action which reduced or even removed the prospects for a coherent, integrated, locally based service, which would address in a holistic manner the needs of disabled people in all the integrally linked areas of their lives, from health and personal support, through housing, education and work.

The management structure introduced into the health board system on foot of the McKinsey Report developed the three main service delivery programmes within the health boards which are now such a familiar part of the landscape of the local health services. Since this structure has formed the essential core of the service delivery system for people with disabilities for several decades, it is appropriate to look critically at its effectiveness as a delivery mechanism.

Insofar as it is reasonable to make judgements based on the reported experience of the service user, then the programme structure of the health boards has fallen short of the expectation that it would provide an integrated, client-centred approach to meeting needs. The problems created in the lives of disabled people by the fragmentation of services, the proliferation of ways of accessing services, and the absence of a clear, simple path through the service delivery system was the single most frequently expressed frustration of people with disabilities who made submissions to the Commission on the Status of People with Disabilities or attended the Commission's consultative seminars. This difficulty was compounded for people by the absence of easily available, clear information about entitlements. These very real and difficult experiences led people to feel that their lives were sometimes turned into a battleground with service providers and administrators. The Commission on Health Funding was one of the many bodies pointing to this systemic linkage between service structures and the experience of the user.

NEED FOR SYSTEMATIC CO-ORDINATION

Co-ordination is about systemic coherence running through the service system from its conception to its delivery. One of the challenges which must be faced is that of making explicit links between stated national values and local programmes, between policy and the design of systems.

The need to develop systems of co-ordination of disability services has been repeatedly referred to in reports, policy documents, and in the pleas of service users who experience the impact of its absence. It is a difficult and complex concept, which would benefit greatly from the development of a theoretical model setting out a framework which would map the essential linkages between systems of policy-making, planning, funding, administrative structures, administrative systems, data gathering and database systems, and service delivery systems, at national, regional and local level, and track the interrelationship of these with the experience of the service user.

Many of the co-ordination problems embedded in the administrative structures of the health services, identified in the report of the Commission on Health Funding and in the report of the National Economic and Social Council on community care (1988), have been taken on board in the Department of Health's strategic framework for future development of the health services (Dept. of Health, 1994). The *Health Strategy* proposes new health legislation which will address the need for decisions about services to be taken as close as possible to the point of delivery. However, the strategy does not give a precise account of how the organisational arrangements within the existing structures might be changed, suggesting that 'the detailed management structure will be worked out at health authority level to ensure that local conditions can be taken into account'.

It will be important for the planners of new structures to take as their starting-point the primary objective of building both administrative and management structures based on a nationally agreed set of values, and an agreed view as to what constitutes excellence in models of service delivery.

MAXIMUM CHOICE AND INDEPENDENCE

As one of its core values, the delivery system needs to provide for maximum choice and independence for people with disabilities, and should optimise the possibility of living within one's community and family. These values or principles are explicit and implicit in virtually every policy document concerning people with disabilities that has been produced in the last twenty-five years. As an administrative goal, the service delivery model should lead to a holistic, seamless continuum of service through which disabled people and families can move with maximum ease at local level. User satisfaction should be a key performance measure, in line with the thrust of the *Health Strategy*, and user participation systems should enable disabled people to influence decisions which materially affect their lives, at both local and national level.

These service values are integral to the idea of community care. As a system of service delivery, it has the potential to promote independence, facilitate choice of service at local level and enable people with disabilities to live within their own community, with the necessary supports. One might argue that, in line with best current thinking, it would now be appropriate to move to using the term 'community support'.

The adoption by the health services of a philosophy of community care, backed up by structures which aim to deliver health and support services based on this philosophy, has been one of the most significant developments during the past fifty years. The 1987 report of the National Economic and Social Council on community care services points out that the emphasis on community care was strong in four major reports produced in the 1960s on mental handicap services, psychiatric services and services for the elderly, and in the White Paper, *The Health Services and their Future Development,* published in 1966. These reports laid the foundation for the formal adoption of the community care concept and the introduction of structures to support it in the 1970 Health Act.

One of the core purposes of the community care structure within the health boards was to build a client-centred, co-ordinated approach to service delivery which would aim to provide support for people with disabilities, the elderly and other vulnerable groups in their local community. The very succinct, comprehensive and conceptually coherent NESC report already referred to outlines the reasons why, in spite of the remarkable level of agreement about the value of community care, the goal had not up to then been translated into a reality. It raised the very pertinent question as to whether, in its working out 'on the ground,' community care tends to substitute for family support rather than to act as a preventive support for the informal family or community network.

This dilemma remains today for people with disabilities. It can have a serious impact on the quality of life of many people with disabilities, as is graphically illustrated in the review of submissions undertaken for the Commission on the Status of People with Disabilities. The data gathering undertaken by the Commission identified as an ongoing problem the unstructured, discretionary nature of many of the most crucial family support services, such as technical and mechanical aids, and a whole range of personal support services. The most flexible personal support services can be disadvantaged by their very informality; the most structured services, which are mainly provided by paid professional staff, tend to have inbuilt mechanisms to ensure continuity and to attract incremental improvements in funding. Well established, formal services have the means and the expertise to utilise to the full opportunities arising from sources of funding such as the range of EU programmes.

The service agreements which are to be a feature of the new voluntary/statutory landscape should not tend to copperfasten this imbalance. While giving the major NGOs the stability which they clearly need, it will be important to find ways of ensuring that their strong prior claim on health board funding does not make even more vulnerable the community-based personal support services which are so crucial to the well-being of disabled people and families. Arrangements such as service brokerage which facilitate choice by people with disabilities and their families require considerable flexibility on the part of service providers.

The NESC Report sums up well the possible tensions between flexibility and structure, and proposes that a real dilemma exists as to 'how to provide a range of services that are flexible enough to meet a variety of needs, and yet allow for structuring and planning.' And with regard to funding, we still need to heed the warning from NESC:

> If expenditures have to be contained it is essential that economies are not distributed solely on the basis of least resistance from service beneficiaries, e.g. in discretionary services.

A LOCAL CONTINUUM OF SERVICE

One of the ways of ensuring balance of provision is through the development of a local continuum of service. The concept of a local continuum of service is a crucial one for people with disabilities and their families. To work effectively, it requires:

* local availability of the 'core' services which people with disabilities need;

* ongoing mechanisms for consultation with people with disabilities about the content of the 'core', and a commitment (legal or strongly formal) to include the core services in the local continuum;

* maximum information about availability of the core services;

* ease of transition from one service to another, even where these are run by different agencies or departments, requiring flexibility of admissions systems and ease of movement into and out of services;

* flexible transport systems;

* speedy, simple systems for determining eligibility;

* a system of ongoing regular review of the individual's needs;

* a support process to enable the individual to negotiate transitions.

The 'pieces' of the continuum are often in place in an area or a region, but the linkages needed to translate that provision into a smooth running continuum are not common.

The Commission on the Status of People with Disabilities has proposed a new infrastructure for services in which the elements of the continuum would be developed at local level. The personal support co-ordinator role envisaged by the Commission is critical to the effective working of the continuum, from the point of view of the service user. People say, very clearly, that they need personal, individualised help to negotiate the service delivery system. The system needs to listen and to respond positively. There is a strong case for piloting such a mechanism, and hearing from the consumer whether it made a difference in their lives.

The service continuum which is described here needs to extend through all community services which support dependence or facilitate independence for disabled people. We need strong models of inter-agency working, supported from the top, possibly through the Government's Strategic Management Initiative.

Local co-ordinating committees have been in place for mental handicap services for some time; the extension of this structure is seen as one of the most important ways of bringing about a coherent, cost-effective local service. Clearly, the effectiveness of the co-ordinating committee structure as a tool to plan to meet local needs, depends on its composition, its brief, its *modus operandi,* the assumptions made by those who participate as to what constitutes an optimal service, and most especially, the mechanisms used to identify need. An overarching regional strategy will be needed, which will transcend the boundaries of provision for the separate disability groupings and identify the potential for sharing resources within communities. That strategy will also need to give an equitable focus to the needs of people with mental health difficulties, people with rare disabilities, women with disabilities and other groups whose needs might not be readily identified through a co-ordinating committee structure.

USER-CENTRED MODEL

The service user is at the heart of the new health strategy which will shape the development of health and personal support services into the 21st century. How are the user's needs to be established? How is the summation of people's needs to be fed into the local planning process? When scarce resources require choices to be made and priorities determined, how are these choices and priorities to be established? Where are the sources of influence? When national level decisions are to be made about the allocation of resources and the expression of that allocation in budgetary policy, how are the users to bring their collective view to bear on this process?

These questions are posed so as to highlight the value-laden nature of daily practices and processes within the service delivery system (a reality which is not of course confined to the services for people with disabilities). Yet these values are rarely made explicit. The systems for the identification and measurement of need, the ways of planning to meet these needs and the ways of checking if these needs have been met at individual, local, regional and national level are the focal points and expressions of the most significant cultural shift taking place in service delivery systems. They are the battleground on which is fought out the tension between the 'expert' model of service and the user-centred model.

At the level of the individual, the user-centred model depends on the development of systems through which people will participate actively in the determination of their own needs, and will in fact lead that process. It will require a sea-change in the attitudes and approach of professionals involved in the assessment process, and a new and less prominent role for medical and paramedical evaluation. These shifts in thinking and in practice will not happen easily. The reality is that the service user cannot lead them. They must be led by the policy-makers and the professionals. They will not be free of cost. New models of self-assessment are being tested and introduced in other jurisdictions. There is a need for health service planners to invest in piloting these models here, and in training staff and users to operate them. People with disabilities and their families need access to advocacy systems and effective complaints procedures as essential mechanisms to enable them to argue their case.

At the local planning level, the user-centred model depends on the introduction of systems to enable people with disabilities to participate fully in local planning committees. The advent of the Council for People with Disabilities should offer a consistent point of access through which disabled people can come forward to join in local planning processes. But the representative structures will not be enough. Meaningful consultation and participation depend on information, and on the provision of supports for those who want to participate. In the absence of these supports, user participation can 'be more concerned with form than content, with rhetoric than reality' (Rafferty, 1996).

NEED FOR DATA

The activity which links personal self-assessment, on the one hand, and the planning process on the other is that of data gathering and database construction. Every report on disability issues and policy that has been produced in the past twenty years in Ireland has expressed concern about the lack of data on disability, for the purpose of planning services.

Databases which attempt to 'log' service need in respect of people with physical and sensory disability cannot be constructed from statistics on incidence or prevalence. The profile of need for one person with, say, cerebral palsy, may be totally different from that of another person with a similar diagnostic profile. There is no intrinsic link between disability category and service need. However, it should be very possible to build profiles of service needs at local level from the consistent and regular use of instruments such as focus groups of people with disabilities in an area, service user audits, small scale qualitative studies carried out in partnership with groups of people with disabilities, carers, families. These instruments can serve the dual purpose of assessing user satisfaction with existing services – thus meeting an objective of the health strategy - while at the same time generating valuable 'bottom-up' data for local planning and ultimately national planning purposes. We must invest in building the skills needed to implement these processes successfully on an ongoing basis. The long-term benefit would be the systematic development of a user-centred health service, engaging in an ongoing process of reviewing and revising services in the light of identified need.

THE ROLE OF REVIEW BODIES AND WORKING PARTIES

By building into our service delivery system flexible user-centred mechanisms for profiling need and planning services, would we reduce the need for working parties, review bodies and commissions, which have been such a significant feature of the landscape within the services for people with disabilities for the past fifty years? While there has not been any systematic examination of the impact of these high level groups on policy and practice, their influence is readily observable. The 1965 *Commission of Enquiry on Mental Handicap*, for example, exerted a very significant influence on all aspects of service structure within mental handicap services; the 1974 *Report on the Training and Employment of the Handicapped* built a structure for the training and vocational development of people with disabilities which embodied radical ideas of full citizenship and independence. The community workshop concept which was a central focus of the proposals offered the chance for disabled trainees to have a genuine continuum of opportunity for vocational development. Significant European funds flowed into Ireland through these new vocational training opportunities, and a major infrastructure of services was created, based on the thinking in this report. It is likely that there will always be a need for such detached, in-depth national appraisals which seek to chart new courses by taking account of cultural change and new thinking in service delivery. For the future, however, it is likely that systems will be in place to facilitate incremental change in response to identified need, in between major policy reviews.

We must expect to see the membership of review bodies and working parties change to reflect our new understanding of the importance of user participation at all levels of the system. The Commission on the Status of People with Disabilities, with 60% of its membership drawn from among the users of services, was in tune with modern thinking and values concerning participatory democracy, equality, and self-determination for people with disabilities. For the future, the thrust for equality of influence for people with disabilities at all levels of the system will surely continue to be reflected in their membership of all agencies and bodies, whether they have a permanent life, such as the new health authorities, or a short term existence as working groups or review bodies.

Perhaps it is this cultural shift towards an equality agenda which has been one of the most significant features of recent decades. Its early manifestations in Ireland in the 1970s and 1980s reflected the growing Independent Living movement in the United States. Under the influence of activists like the late Liam Maguire, the access programme was given a strong impetus. A committed trade unionist, Liam succeeded in placing disability issues firmly on the agenda of the Irish Congress of Trade Unions, and that success has had a very significant impact to the present day. It has ensured, for example, that disability issues have featured strongly in successive national agreements. The Forum of People with Disabilities was the first organisation made up solely of people with disabilities, speaking for people with disabilities. It was influential in the setting up of the Commission on the Status of People with Disabilities, and secured a commitment for the setting up of a permanent Council for the Status of People with Disabilities. That Council is now in place and has secured a reasonably substantial budget for its activities.

INFLUENCE OF INTERNATIONAL BODIES

The movement towards a civil rights focus on disability issues, with its emphasis on legislative provision for equality and full participation, draws heavily on international models and the support of respected and influential international bodies. The Americans with Disabilities Act, which consolidated and extended legislative provision for anti-discrimination measures in the

United States, is serving as a model for anti-discrimination legislation in other parts of the world, including Ireland, where the Commission on the Status of People with Disabilities has made proposals for a Disabilities Act. Perhaps the most powerful measure which will move us towards the implementation of an equality agenda for people with disabilities, in all aspects of living as well as health services, is the UN Standard Rules on the Equalisation of Opportunities for Persons with Disabilities, adopted by the United Nations in 1993. Although not legally binding on UN member states, these Rules provide a legal standard for programmes, policies and laws which address the issue of full participation and equality for people with disabilities. They are of immense significance in that they provide specific targets for participation across the spectrum of aspects of daily living, thus offering ready-made performance indicators for any government seriously committed to the task of securing inclusion and participation. The Rules underpin the partnership agreement between the Department of Health and the Federation of Voluntary Organisations providing services for people with mental handicap. In the European Union context, their significance is heightened now because the Rules have been built into a Resolution of the European Union and the Council, adopted in December 1996.

SUMMING UP

The extent of the development of health and personal support services for people with disabilities over the past fifty years has been remarkable in its range and scope. Expenditure on disability services has increased almost tenfold in the past twenty years alone, from £26 million in 1975 to over £220 million in 1995. This figure does not take account of the cost of the range of income maintenance services or the cost of the psychiatric services, which itself amounted to over £200 million in 1993. While this increase is accounted for in part by inflationary pressures, and switches from privately-funded to publicly-funded service provision, nonetheless there has been an obvious increase in the volume and extent of services. The commitment of successive governments and administrations to the development of services is clearly strong and continuing.

How might one sum up the past fifty years and anticipate the future of health and personal support services for people with disabilities and their families? The last half decade has been one of significant growth in the scale and sophistication of services, in particular for people with learning difficulties or mental handicap; a legislative framework has been established; national and local structures for service delivery have emerged. The health board system, in partnership with the voluntary sector, has facilitated the development of local responses to local need, innovation and experimentation. We have a sound foundation of services on which to build new models of service responsive to the changing culture which will characterise the new millennium.

The culture of care which has so strongly characterised the past fifty years must be balanced for the future by the development of a culture of formal support for independence. The tools of the systems of service delivery must be recast so that the service user gains influence and control over the decisions at local, regional and national level that shape her daily life. The professional service provider must refashion the systems of assessment, of decision-making, of planning and prioritising, to allow for a new relationship of respect with the service users who are expert in their own lives and their own needs.

The agenda of equality must merge with the service delivery agenda, to fashion new partnerships. At the policy-making level this will require a strong, successful partnership between the Department of Equality and Law Reform and the main service-providing departments, including the Department of Health. New structures such as the National Disability Authority proposed by the Commission on the Status of People with Disabilities will be needed to assist in the task of setting equality targets, developing measures of successful outcomes from a user perspective, supporting participation in its many facets and monitoring progress towards a fair and equitable society in which disabled people can have real choices, and make those choices themselves. The climate is right for these shifts of focus, if the structures can be sufficiently responsive to enable and support change.

The challenge will be one of retaining or even regaining balance; in terms of both quality and quantity of services, many would argue that there has been an imbalance in investment in different groups of disabled people, and that we now need a new focus – particularly on those with behavioural difficulties, with neurological problems, with mental health difficulties.

We need to retain the balance, too, between a rights agenda and the need to maintain a place for caring and supportive local communities who can and should carry a shared responsibility for and interest in the welfare and well-being of all their members:

> neither human existence nor individual liberty can be sustained for long outside the interdependent and overlapping communities to which we all belong. Nor can any community long survive unless its members dedicate some of their energy, attention and resources to shared projects (Etzioni, 1993).

It would be ironic indeed if in the future the understandable desire to move from dependence on charity and goodwill to entitlement as of right were to increase the dependence of people with disabilities on professional service providers, and lessen the role of supportive family and community. It would be a pity if, in the task of changing the language of discourse about disability to one which is more respectful, we were to inadvertently label disabled people all over again with new politically correct labels, but labels nonetheless. It would be understandable if the process of setting up structures of influence for people with disabilities were to create new hierarchies and new ghettos. We must take care to maintain all these delicate balances as we build the future on the solid foundation of the past. The biggest difference may be that disabled people themselves can be the architects, planners and builders of that future and not simply the passive inhabitants of it.

CHAPTER 10

Mental Health Care in Ireland 1945-1997 and the Future

Dermot Walsh

Although the Department of Health came into being in 1947, it is appropriate to begin this review two years earlier, in 1945, because this year was significant for the delivery of mental health care in Ireland. It saw the introduction of the Mental Treatment Act (1945) which replaced the lunacy laws of the earlier part of the century.

There are a few dates in history that can be thought of as definitive, for example the fall of Constantinople in May 1453, and all that that implied for the future of European civilisation. Similarly, 31 December 1958 marked the summit of mental hospital care in Ireland. On that day 21,046 patients were returned as inhabiting district mental hospitals, approximately 0.5% of the Irish population. Not that this represented the acme of institutionalisation; that accolade went to St. Columba's Hospital in Sligo which in the same year accommodated almost 800 patients, representing 0.7% of the Sligo/Leitrim catchment area. This then was the final vindication of Victorian policy in relation to the indigent mentally ill who, of course, comprised the majority. Successive reports of the inspectors of lunacy addressed the 'apparent' increase in lunacy (whether it was real or artefactual was never conclusively decided) and the necessity of providing additional asylum care and of implementing a policy of transferring lunatics 'at large', in workhouses, bridewells and in jails to appropriate accommodation in district lunatic asylums. Concomitantly, from 1840 onwards another section of indigent poor had been accommodated under a system of indoor relief in the workhouses. Even though the two systems were identified as dealing with two different streams of disability, there was a good deal of overlap.

The first half of the twentieth century was largely a time of consolidation and retrenchment, with the only notable frisson in an unchanged and unchanging scene being the separation of the district asylums of the Northern six counties from those of the emergent Irish Free State in 1922. Generally asylums had become independent entities, walled off from the communities which they served, with an extensive range of provision for everyday living within their precincts, resembling a medieval fortress town. The intra-mural residential accommodation for patients and staff at all levels guaranteed the preservation of the asylum just as surely as the walls built by Constantine and Justinian protected Byzantium. But, just as Constantinople was to fall, so the asylum system was less secure than it believed in the 1920s and 1930s. Yet the lunatic asylum or mental hospital was as vital to its community as it was separate from it. The 1951 census of population of the town of Ballinasloe, in which the Connaught Asylum was opened in the year 1833, returned a population of 5,596 persons. Of these 2,078 were patients in the mental hospital, which the asylum had now become, and 439 were full-time employees of the hospital. In addition, there can be little doubt that the townspeople derived some economic benefit, direct or indirect, from the existence of the institution. In the days before the IDA brought industry to the towns of Ireland, the hospital system provided occupational opportunity, allowing some employees to work, marry and withstand emigration.

1945 AND ALL THAT

The most important provision of the 1945 Mental Treatment Act was the introduction of the category of 'voluntary' patient. This enabled persons to enter psychiatric or mental hospitals of their own free will, presumably in the belief that persons could realise that they were mentally ill and seek treatment for that illness, whereas previously the consensus was that anyone who pursued such a course of action was deemed thereby to be in need of certification. It was 1947 before the Act came into operation, and in that year the first voluntary patients crossed mental hospital thresholds. By the end of the year, 376 out of a total of 3,700 admissions were voluntary, and it was noted that there had been a considerable increase in admissions overall in the years following the introduction of the new legislation. At the end of 1947, of the 17,791 patients resident in district and auxiliary mental hospitals 114 were voluntary; and of the 882 patients in private, charitable and authorised mental institutions, 304 were voluntary, indicating a much greater up-take of this new admission category by private compared to public hospitals. On a more general note, of the 2,544 receptions or admissions in 1946, 2,055 were returned as first admissions.

Another step forward in legislation and practice was the provision whereby involuntary patients were allowed out on 'absence on trial'. In 1947 this facility was accorded to 648 patients. The rationale behind the provision was that if the patients allowed out satisfied all concerned that their illness had improved sufficiently, they would then be discharged. If, on the other hand, their condition deteriorated, they could be returned to hospital without any formality; they did not have to be recertified.

The average cost per year of maintaining a patient had risen from £59 in 1941 to over double this, £118, by 1948. Each hospital had its farm, and the total acreage of district mental hospital land, most of which was farmed, amounted to just under 7,000, varying from a total of 991 acres at St Ita's, Portrane to 135 at St Davnet's, Monaghan. The expenditure on capital works in the mental hospitals of Ireland up to the end of 1948, with payments being made from the Hospitals Trust Fund, amounted to £1,195,383. This sum was spent on a diversity of provisions ranging from nurses' homes to refrigerators and the installation of new boilers. However, the annual expenditure was somewhat less impressive, working out for the year 1949 as £30,000. The essentially structural, particularly agricultural, nature of the destination of some of this expenditure can be appreciated by the provision of a new corn loft and a new potato storage shed at Ardee and a new piggery at Waterford.

Persons flooded to the psychiatric hospitals in this era, just as they had done in the nineteenth century. Once a person was directed towards a mental hospital, no bar to reception or admission was placed in his way. Indeed, since the senior staff members were remunerated in accordance with the number of beds under their control, it became vital in the larger hospitals to ensure that this number did not dip below 1,000. The openness of the mental hospital system did not pass unnoticed by those seeking accommodation for a variety of miscellaneous problems in the outside world. Whatever about the inappropriateness of confinement of children, the elderly, the socially marginalised and particularly the mentally handicapped, these all flooded in, to the evident relief of the community, families and other institutions, if not to the individuals themselves. In 1963 no less than sixteen per cent of the occupants of Irish psychiatric hospitals were there not because they were mentally ill, but because they were mentally handicapped, many of them having found their way via the more selective institutions for this condition run by voluntary agencies.

All hospitals consisted of a male and a female 'house' and male and female patients seldom mixed, except occasionally at recreational facilities such as dances in the hospital's recreation hall. The 1945 Act was specific in maintaining separate gender arrangements within hospitals to ensure that no moral affront or outrage should be added to the stigma that the mentally ill, even in their residential and institutionalised settings, suffered. In a general sense, it was believed that work made persons free of their illness, or at least helped to alleviate it. This precept had been recognised since the era of moral treatment in mental illness in the nineteenth century and it was reaffirmed in the more active psychiatric hospitals in the 1950s. Indeed, one medical superintendent wrote a book on occupational therapy.

The mental hospitals were run hierarchically, with the resident medical superintendent reporting to the mental hospital board. This existed independently of any other health administrative unit, although this was to change with the setting up in the 1960s of 'composite' health authorities and later, of course, with the inauguration of health boards in 1970, with global responsibility for health and social care. The medical superintendent was autonomous and autocratic, his authority being supported by that of one or more senior assistant medical officers who in turn were helped by assistant medical officers of a more junior standing. Attendants, attired in constabulary-like uniforms for the males, with aprons and caps for the women, were edging towards respectability, and the change from attendant to nurse was not far away. In the mid-1950s a very small number of general trained nurses were imported into the mental hospital system and utilised for the more technical nursing procedures.

Treatments, too, were beginning to evolve. Up to the middle 1950s there was little available by way of specific medical treatment for psychiatric disorders, although many imaginative procedures had been tried without enduring effect, other than in the consciousness of those who had been exposed to them. In the 1950s, for instance, convulsive therapy was introduced and given 'straight', i.e. patients were neither anaesthetised nor were they given muscle relaxants to ensure that the ensuing convulsion, electrically administered, was not too violent. Whatever about the improvement in their mental state (and some depressives did undoubtedly improve following this treatment) the toll of broken and dislocated bones and aching muscles was appreciable.

In the 1950s and into the 1960s, insulin coma therapy for first onset schizophrenic patients was all the vogue. Such patients were rendered comatose by the administration of insulin, which brought down their blood sugar levels and sent them into a coma from which they were released by the administration of glucose. Most woke up within half an hour; very occasionally some obstinate ones refused to oblige, at which stage the coma was designated 'irreversible' and, despite heroic intravenous administration of glucose, some patients died. Later in the 1960s, controlled clinical trials showed unequivocally that any benefit that derived from this treatment was not directly attributable to the induced coma but rather to the social and 'moral' aspects of the treatment associated with it.

Brain surgery or leucotomy was hailed as a new therapeutic marvel and selected cases were chosen for this procedure. Unfortunately, some of the results were not encouraging, either because of their side effects, which could be quite disabling, or because no clinical improvement in mental state ensued. In the 1960s this treatment, like insulin-coma treatment, was beginning to lose favour and declined in usage, although it still lingers to a very small extent in highly selected cases to this day. The administration of electro-convulsive therapy (ECT) became more refined in its minutiae and into the 1960s patients were anaesthetised and given muscle relaxants to ensure that the less pleasant aspects of 'straight' ECT were eliminated. If the 1950s was the 'heroic' age of experimental treatment in psychiatry, then the 1960s was the era of 'modified' ECT with very few patients coming to mental hospitals escaping its administration at one time or another. In the larger hospitals, such as St Brendan's, it was not uncommon for fifty to sixty patients to be on the ECT lists on treatment days.

The late 1950s were heroic in another treatment sense, and that was the introduction of psychotrophic drugs. These were drugs for depression, and tranquillising and sedative drugs. By the early 1960s both categories of drugs were in widespread use, and so they continue to this day.

CHANGE AND PROGRESS

It had not gone unnoticed that the numbers of patients in Irish psychiatric hospitals and their proportion relative to the general population was higher than anywhere else in the world. This was a matter for concern, not alone for the national image, but also because, being approximately twice that of neighbouring countries, there were implications for the cost of running the mental health service. Large numbers were kept in confined areas in hospitals, with some wards containing up to 120 patients living in poor conditions. This forced government action and the setting up of a Commission of Inquiry on Mental Illness in 1961. This commission was representative of most walks of Irish life as well as the Irish professional psychiatric interest, reinforced by some professional figures of consequence from Britain. The terms of reference were to:

–   examine and report on the health services available for the mentally ill and make recommendations on the most practicable and desirable measures for the improvement of these services

–   consider and report on changes regarded as necessary or desirable in the legislation dealing with the mentally ill.

The Commission produced its report in 1966. The main thrust of the report was that Irish psychiatric services were very institutionalised and that, apart from out-patient clinics, little was available by way of service and treatment alternatives to hospitalisation. It recommended that patient care for the future should be provided in small psychiatric units in general hospitals and that there should be a movement away from the large, isolated, institutionalising mental hospital. It also recommended a variety of community-based alternatives, such as day hospitals, day centres, hostels and community-based residences. It recommended the employment of multi-disciplinary teams to deal with psychiatric illness, so that social workers, psychologists, occupational therapists and others should be recruited to the service which up until then had relied exclusively on doctors and nurses. It advised a much greater participation of general practitioners in mental health care, and advocated the setting up and development of child psychiatric services which up to this point scarcely existed, apart from one or two initiatives in the Dublin area. The Commission was ingenuous enough to suggest that if its recommendations were implemented the number of beds necessary to deal with psychiatric illness would fall in fifteen years' time (i.e. in 1981) by over half, to 8,000.

Undoubtedly the Commission's report was of high quality and its recommendations were soundly based. However, its major shortcoming was that it did not discuss or advise on how these might be implemented or progressed. The consequences were that no formal processes for implementation eventuated, either nationally or locally. It is nonetheless true that individual initiatives appeared sporadically, and geographically unevenly, throughout the country. Thus in 1965 the first psychiatric unit in a general hospital was established in Ardkeen Hospital in Waterford. Outpatient clinics were provided in some general hospitals and health centres, and a plan was drawn up to decentralise the health services in the Dublin area. These hitherto had been centrally based at St Brendan's Hospital in Grangegorman, with an auxiliary hospital dating from the turn of the century at St Ita's in Portrane. The main stimulus to decentralisation was probably the acquisition by the Dublin Health Authority of a former sanatorium at Ballyowen in West County Dublin, which had been purpose built and opened in the 1950s, but never fully occupied and closed shortly afterwards. It was given to the mental health services and after a period of dependency on St Brendan's, having opened in 1961, became autonomous and began to serve a catchment area in West Dublin in 1966. This redundant institutional over-provision for tuberculosis was echoed throughout the country, and further sanatoria became available to the psychiatric services elsewhere in the country.

The planning of mental health services in the Dublin area was based on the principle of decentralisation and continuity of care, providing a comprehensive service that was multi-disciplinary and integrated with primary care. Such delivery could only be established on a geographic basis and so the principle of sectorisation, borrowed from francophone psychiatry, became, by 1971, the basis of care delivery in what became the Eastern Health Board area. Decentralisation to establish independent geographically local services was pursued, and clinical directors were appointed to head up each local service. In-patient units for each local catchment area were eagerly sought and opened.

PLANNING FOR THE FUTURE

Despite all this flurry of activity, particularly on the east coast, by 1981 the Commission's predictions were far from being fulfilled, with the number of patients not just reaching the projected 8,000 but approximately twice this number. Accordingly it was felt necessary to set up another body to assess the existing service, to clarify objectives and to draw up planning guidelines for future developmen. The brief given to the Study Group appointed by the Minister for Health, Eileen Desmond TD, in October 1981 flowed from the perception that insufficient progress had been made in implementing the Commission's report, and that the time was ripe for inpatient treatment for all admissions to be provided in psychiatric units in general hospitals.

The Study Group's findings were set out in *Planning for the Future,* published in 1984. The Group envisaged a service that was comprehensive, community orientated, sectorised and integrated. It stressed the need for provision of community-based physical resources to provide community-based residential care and day care. It stressed also the need to rehabilitate the existing long-stay patients in psychiatric hospitals so that they would be relieved of their disabilities and handicaps to the extent that they would be capable of living normal community lives once again, and the need for specialisation in this particular area. It identified the elderly mentally infirm as a separate category of patient for whom 'in densely populated areas' a dedicated psychiatric team, led by a psychiatrist, would specialise in dealing with the psychiatry of later life. *Planning for the Future* specifically recommended that patients suffering from dementia should not be routinely cared for by the psychiatric services. It stressed too that assessment of the elderly psychiatrically infirm should be undertaken in community-based settings or in primary care.

Another group considered by the report was that of substance abuse-related patients, and it was critical of the predominantly psychiatric hospitalised approach to this problem which had resulted in one-third of male admissions to psychiatric hospitals being for alcohol-related problems. While deploring the lack of community-based preventive action for alcohol problems, the report suggested that psychiatric services should develop sector-based and community-based local alcoholism services, and advised that 'one consultant psychiatrist take responsibility for the organisation and operation of services for persons with alcohol related problems in the area'. In relation to drug problems other than alcohol, the report favoured community intervention rather than general practitioner involvement in treatment. Finally, attention was given to the urgency of extending child psychiatric services throughout the country.

Unlike its predecessor, the Commission of Inquiry Report in 1966, *Planning for the Future*, devoted separate chapters to the organisation and management of psychiatric services at local level. It also reviewed cost implications and suggested that in providing psychiatric units in general hospitals with a total of 1,700 beds, of approximately 50 beds each per 100,000 of population, the cost would be £34 million. A similar number of places would be necessary for new long-stay psychiatric patients at the somewhat lower cost of £25 million. Day facilities were to be provided (i.e. day hospital and day centre places) at a rate of 0.75 day places per 1,000 of population, creating nationally 2,600 places, bearing in mind that 1,180 places were currently available. This left a shortfall of 1,420 day places which could be provided for at a cost of £8 million. Similarly, community residential places would need to be provided to augment the existing 950 places available in various types of hostels throughout the country. These should be provided, the report felt, through rental arrangements of suitable accommodation and it was the view of the group that £50 million, spread over a ten- to fifteen-year period, would suffice to provide the new service designed along the triad of short-stay psychiatric inpatient units in general hospitals, continuing care residential provision and community-based accommodation involving day places in day hospitals and day centres. This contrasted with an estimate of £150 million if reliance were to be exclusively on existing psychiatric hospital accommodation in buildings brought up to acceptable modern standards. *Planning for the Future* was in no doubt as to which of these two options was the more desirable. It felt that the revenues currently being provided to the psychiatric service need not be increased for the new service envisaged in its report.

THE RESPONSE

Progress on the implementation of the recommendations of planning for the future was reviewed by the *Green Paper on Mental Health 1992*. Because of the attention to consideration of planning and implementation, it was certainly true to say that *Planning for the Future* made a much greater impact on psychiatric services and those who worked in them and planned for them, both at central and local level, than was the case of the *Report of the Commission of Inquiry on Mental Illness*, excellent though that report was. Management and planning groups were set up in most psychiatric services, sectorisation was pursued and effected throughout the country with few exceptions, these, curiously enough, being for the most part in psychiatric services which also served an academic function. In the meantime bed numbers continued to fall and the provision of psychiatric units in general hospitals continued to grow, so that by the end of 1996 sixteen units existed throughout the country and many more were at planning stage. Numbers in psychiatric hospitals declined largely through mortality of former long-stay patients, and those remaining behind grew increasingly old, so that more than 50% of long-stay patients by the end of 1996 were sixty-five or over and a third were seventy-five or over. At the other end the rate of accumulation of new long-stay patients had dropped away considerably, that is patients passing from under to over one year of continuous inpatient care. With a rate of decrement far greater then that of their replacement, all the indications were that in another fifteen years the long-stay hospital population would have ceased to exist. Indeed in some instances former mental hospitals had been sold, as in Sligo and Cork. In other locations large tracts of former mental hospital wards were empty and unoccupied, although some had been turned to alternative usage such as St Mary's, Castlebar, where a greater part of the hospital was now serving as a modern third-level educational college. By the end of 1995, the total resident population in psychiatric hospitals, public and private and in psychiatric general hospital units, was 5,830.

Mental health centres or sector headquarters providing the community base for the multi-disciplinary sector psychiatric team were being established throughout the country. By the end of 1996 this exercise was complete in many services and was ongoing in others. Thus, in line with good health care delivery practice, the majority of mental health services were now available to individuals in their own communities and near their own homes, with a corresponding de-emphasising of the inpatient base. Professionals had now passed the psychological barrier of movement from institution to community by recognising the mental health centre as a major and predominating work location, claiming their travelling expenses from it rather than from the inpatient base. Most mental health centres either provided active day hospital facilities within their fabric or had them close by. Thus primary care sources were learning, albeit slowly in some instances, to refer cases for psychiatric assessment to mental health centres rather than to psychiatric or general hospitals. Community residential places began to increase in hostels, group homes and so on. The rate of rehabilitation of long-stay in-patients from hospitals to community residences, and in some cases, for the more disabled persons, to high support hostels, increased greatly. By now the 'gold standard' of care provision had begun to change. The inpatient provision had dropped to something of the order of 35 acute inpatient beds per 100,000 of population with a corresponding increase to 1 or 1.5 per 100,000 of population, for day and community-based residential places. At the same time there was recognition that secure treatment facilities were necessary for a very small handful of patients not deemed manageable in the 'ordinary' residential treatment facilities, and in 1995 the Department of Health set up a special task force to advise it on what was necessary in this regard.

PRIVATE HOSPITALS

The numbers of private services reduced, with two main services, based in Dublin, providing most of the acute care. Both St Patrick's Hospital and St John of God's Hospital were, by the end of 1996, functioning as traditional psychiatric hospitals. Both provided comfortable, high quality inpatient accommodation and treatment for patients financially supported by the Voluntary Health Insurance organisation and other insurance schemes. The substantial class division between the public and private services was exemplified by the social status of patients of the two major groups, public and private, although the provision of psychiatric units in general hospitals was, in small measure, tending to attract, in local areas, patients from a social background hitherto unlikely to avail of public services. With increasing competitiveness in the private health care insurance market, particularly a decrease in the length of inpatient cover, private hospitals were looking in the direction of providing specialised inpatient care for all sections of the community, and attempting to extend the range of their services beyond the inpatient level. At the same time, the two major hospitals had joined with the public service in providing, on a contract basis, area psychiatric services for the Eastern Health Board. In the case of St John of God's Hospital this was logical enough, as this was a service with an inpatient base in the private hospital as well as being the provider of services from a free-standing community-based headquarters. In the case of St Patrick's the situation was more complicated in that this hospital was responsible for running the community service of the St James's Hospital public psychiatric service. The inpatient base was a fifty-bed unit based in that hospital.

THE MENTAL HOSPITAL INSPECTORATE

As obliged by statute the inspectorate of mental hospitals continued throughout this period to be responsible for overseeing standards of care and other relevant matters in psychiatric services. Annual reports of the inspectorate to the Minister for Health continued to give an overview of mental health services in the country. These reports were complemented by statistical information on a range of medical and socio-demographic parameters supplied on an annual basis on inpatient services by the Medico-Social Research Board and later its successor, the Health Research Board. These data on in-patient activity were supplemented by the establishment of psychiatric case registers, providing longitudinal information on patient movement throughout all phases of psychiatric care.

MENTAL HEALTH LEGISLATION

The Commission of Enquiry on Mental Illness, while acknowledging that the Mental Treatment Act 1945 was a fundamentally progressive and sound piece of legislation for its time, believed it needed replacement. Accordingly in 1981 the Health (Mental Services) Act was passed by the Oireachtas, but was not brought into operation because of a number of considerations, including some technical flaws. A substantial part of the *Green Paper on Mental Health 1992* indicated a commitment to creating new legislation and indicated what the main thrust of that legislation would be. It centred on several statements of principle by international bodies such as the United Nations and it stressed the importance of the civil rights of the mentally ill. To ensure that these were protected it was of the view that a central autonomous statutory body, to be known as the Mental Health Review Board, should be set up and would have, along with other specific duties, that of independently reviewing every involuntary admission to psychiatric centres, and through regional panels allowing an extensive appeals mechanism to be put in place. Among its proposed provisions the new legislation would introduce informal admission, would reduce the duration of involuntary admission, and would, on an annual basis, review each and every case of involuntary detention. It saw the review role of the Inspector of Mental Hospitals being taken over by the Mental Health Review Board and felt that the quality assurance role of that post should continue through the role of Commissioner of Mental Health. This would replace that of the Inspector of Mental Hospitals. On balance it was of the view that the post of clinical director (the successor to the resident medical superintendent) of mental health services should continue to be a statutory one, although it favoured a rotation of the post among consultant psychiatrists on a fixed term basis. Having taken full account of a large number of submissions and the views of interested bodies, the Department of Health published in 1995 a subsequent *White Paper on Mental Health Legislation,* and the proposals therein have been followed by the heads of a bill which is now the subject of drafting.

THE FUTURE

Psychiatric care in Ireland, as elsewhere, is now headed irrevocably towards comprehensive, integrated high quality community care. The fate of the large mental hospital is sealed and by the year 2005, at the latest, virtually all acute psychiatric in-patient care will be delivered in psychiatric units in general hospitals. As it is, in 1996, every catchment area service in the country either has a unit in a general hospital or is planning such a unit. Meantime, mental hospitals continue to die. Some are sold, all are partly empty and some have already adapted to other uses, mainly in the education sphere. I have outlined but not completely explained these developments earlier in this chapter. Policy and its implementation has been partly responsible but other forces poorly comprehended have also been at work. Hence, from the late 1950s, sociological forces not fully understood have operated in moving against the institutional containment of the mentally ill. There is, for example, some evidence, by no means conclusive, that serious mental illness is on the decline and that the outlook for its outcome is better than it was in the nineteenth century for reasons that are, again, poorly understood. More powerful (and more expensive) newly-introduced drugs may also be making their contribution to the decline in the need for prolonged hospitalisation, but their influence needs further time, experience and exposure before it can be properly evaluated. Scientific advances in our understanding of the causes of mental illness are slow to come by, but technological advances in neurophysiology and in molecular biology technology, which is set to increase our knowledge of the genetic contribution to major illness, bode well for the future.

SPECIALISED PSYCHIATRIC SERVICES

Meanwhile planning had been going on to improve the psychiatric services available to the criminal justice system and to raise the level of care available in the Central Mental Hospital at Dundrum. By the end of 1996 two new modern units had been opened in the Central Mental Hospital and the number of patients there had fallen by almost one half from the figure of the 1950s. Improvement in the rate of growth of child psychiatric services was less impressive. Nonetheless, progress was reported with specialised child psychiatric services being in place at half a dozen locations outside Dublin by the end of 1966 and with others at the planning stage. Likewise there was a recognition of the need for specialised psychiatric provision for more elderly citizens through the provision of consultant-led psychiatric services specialising in their care. Improvement in the care for the elderly through this development was evidenced as much by improved administrative arrangements as by specific clinical inputs. The community deployment of services for alcohol abuse, although still based in psychiatric services in many instances, was beginning to move towards more direct contact with community service agencies such as general practice. The elimination of admission of mentally handicapped persons to psychiatric inpatient services on the grounds of mental handicap alone was virtually complete. Overall, the last thirty years have seen a considerable refinement emerge in psychiatric services with the honing of provision to match need and the consequent improvement in service delivery to specifically identified target groups in place of the omnibus, asset-wasting approach of the past.

SECTORISATION AND SPECIALISATION

The cornerstone of care delivery today is sectorisation, world-wide and rightly so. However, sectorisation has to learn to co-exist with an increasing thrust towards specialisation. Specialisation within psychiatry, particularly for the young and the elderly, the adolescent or liaison psychiatry within general hospitals, is on the increase and is basically a sound concept. It must be remembered that full-time liaison work may offend the geographic principle and involve discontinuity of care. On the other hand the larger general hospital with multiple tertiary referral units may legitimately seek a specialised psychiatric input which will help staff to deal with the specific psychological problems arising in their units. In this regard the liaison team will have training and consultative functions. These are necessary developments, if only because they represent a more efficient way of dealing with particular problems than currently exists and perhaps determine a better clinical outcome. Nevertheless, there are fears that psychiatry may become too fragmented by specialisation and that a situation comparable to that which currently exists in medicine and surgery, and which is inappropriate outside large metropolises, may strangle the rational development of psychiatric services in Ireland. The psychiatric generalist must still emerge as the cornerstone of a psychiatric service. Some of the problems presenting to psychiatric services currently are not essentially medical and can be equally well, and more cost effectively and efficiently, dealt with by non-medical professionals working in partnership and consultation with psychiatrists. Here it is appropriate to point out that despite the recommendations of *Planning for the Future,* professionals other than doctors and nurses, such as social workers, psychologists, and occupational therapists are still in short supply in mental health services.

PRIMARY CARE AND PSYCHIATRY

All Irish policy documents from the *Report of the Commission of Enquiry on Mental Illness* onwards envisage a far greater participation of primary care in the management of psychiatric illness, even severe illness. Realistically it is doubtful if this situation will change until the structure of primary care in Ireland itself evolves. When sixty per cent of general practices are single-handed, as is currently the case, it is difficult to visualise any greater participation of general practice in the management of what are often complex and multi-faceted conditions with corresponding needs, particularly for the more severe and complex illnesses. The temptation of psychiatry to 'take over' the primary carers' management of patients must be resisted. This is not to say that the contribution of psychiatric specialist consultation to primary care should be diminished. The strengthening of group practices by the availability of community care-based psychologists on the one hand and the increased availability of psychiatric consultation on the other is to be welcomed. When and if primary care develops in the manner suggested, it is inevitable that specialisation in general practice will increase. In this context, it may be envisaged that every general practice will have among its number a doctor with a special interest in psychiatric problems, to whom his fellow general practitioners of the group will likely refer particular cases.

ACADEMIC PSYCHIATRY AND TRAINING

While teaching and research are essential elements of psychiatric services and of teaching general hospitals in particular, it must always be borne in mind that these are means to an end rather than the end itself. The strengthening of the academic base of psychiatry for post graduate teaching purposes including research is essential. Already some strides have been made in this direction, but the combination post of professor of psychiatry and clinical director has helped neither. The case for full-time professorships in psychiatry with a limited clinical load is overwhelming. It is important that Irish postgraduate psychiatric education be regionalised at university and professorial levels, and that postgraduate rotations be put in place.

Some will regret that psychiatry in Ireland, alone of the medical specialities, has not yet evolved its own training programme and accreditation scheme in postgraduate psychiatry, tailored to national cultural and administrative needs, but depends instead on the British Royal College. The number of Irish medical graduates undergoing postgraduate psychiatric training in Ireland, the United Kingdom and to a lesser extent in the USA is substantial, and greater than that needed to fill consultant post vacancies at home. As opportunities for higher training in this country are limited in comparison to the United Kingdom, qualified Irish doctors wishing to train in psychiatry often enter training schemes in the United Kingdom where access is easier, leaving some Irish psychiatric services staffed, at junior medical level, by non-nationals. An expansion of higher training posts and the shortening of postgraduate psychiatric training promise a partial solution to this problem. Indeed, the merging of so-called basic and higher professional training in medical specialities has been urged in the United Kingdom itself. Some of the anxieties responsible for our reluctance to establish an indigenous training and examination system may stem from apprehension that psychiatrists trained in our scheme, had we one, would not have practice reciprocity in the United Kingdom. However, future EU legislation will likely lead to further harmonisation in medical training between EU countries. Already steps have been taken in determining that each national competent authority awards a certificate of completion of specialist training recognised in all EU countries.

As far as nurse training is concerned, there are some anomalies. Psychiatric nurses do not share common training with general nurses. Psychiatric nurse training does not lead to general nurse training qualifications, although most nurses working in psychiatric services are doubly trained as general and psychiatric nurses. On the other hand, general nurses do not have specific psychiatric training, and are not therefore legally recognised as psychiatric nurses.

CONCLUSION

The possibility of the fragmentation of administrative responsibility for psychiatric care between a number of various bodies, which has happened in other jurisdictions, so that hospital care is divorced from community care is a constant apprehension of those working in mental health. Above all, Irish psychiatric services must stand firm on the unified approach. Currently the local delivery and funding of psychiatric care in Ireland is based on programmes specific to it. More recently suggested developments, particularly in the Eastern Health Board Area, must ensure that all health and social services are delivered on a geographic basis, with a specific programme and dedicated budget being available for psychiatry. A more generic and competitive situation, because of the weakness of psychiatry politically, may work against adequate funding for the speciality.

It must be remembered that the mentally ill are in many respects, together with the elderly and the mentally handicapped, the most vulnerable persons in our society. Mental illness is as genuine and real as, and perhaps more damaging than, physical illness. Our health strategy documents have emphasised equity as a cardinal principle of health care delivery. This means equal and just treatment for the mentally ill with the physically ill and between the social classes. Even more importantly is the recognition that among the mentally ill themselves, some handicaps, impairments and disabilities are greater than others, such as those suffering from more serious and personality-eroding illnesses. These persons must not be neglected in the search for a more 'glamorous' psychiatry which deviates scarce resources from their care in the quest for newer and more refined psychiatric empires of conquest. None the less, improvements in the quality of psychiatric care that we deliver are not going to be cheaply bought. Increased specialisation in psychiatry, now almost inevitable, and the capital costs of new general hospital psychiatric units, together with the provision of those community-based physical resources still lacking despite the substantial achievements of recent years, imply a substantial financial burden for the years ahead.

CHAPTER 11

Counselling and the Health Services

Brion Sweeney

One of the newer elements in our health service and one for which there is increasing demand is counselling in various forms. This article looks at the reasons for this development, describes the various types of counselling that have emerged and discusses the need for the setting of standards.

More and more nowadays people are questioning the essence of counselling. Kings and queens of old had counsellors. A counsellor would advise the monarch or help to explore various options in relation to important decisions, but the monarch held the right to make the final decisions that affected the realm. In fact a good counsellor, or at least one who kept his head, would be sure not to make decisions! Later the term counsellor was used to denote legal advice and guidance. The verb to counsel comes from the Latin 'consulo' – to deliberate, take thought, look after, consult the interests of – hence the Roman council and councillors.

What then have been the influences which have changed the prerogative of kings and queens into something that each member of our society sees as a right? It could be said that the demand for counselling is rooted in the emancipation of the individual which has continued apace since the Magna Carta, signed in June 1215, proclaimed fundamental rights of citizenship. In essence today's citizens are seen to be sovereigns of their world, that is, we retain the right to make the crucial decisions in our lives. We also expect to have the same access to a process to assist us in that endeavour as the monarchs of old, i.e. counselling.

Other influences have contributed to the increased demand for counselling. In particular, urbanisation and the move away from small village life have changed the access that we have to the wiser and older within the community. In the past we lived in an extended family where there was ready experience and advice from older members. Some of these possessed a degree of wisdom and perhaps skill in counselling. These skills would have been acquired informally, over time, and may have come down to such observations as the pointlessness of advising someone to do any one thing – people will almost invariably, and rightly, make their own decisions anyway.

Other functions of traditional societies have also been lost. Time to grieve is no longer provided with liberal doses of music, song and poetry, to help memory recall and emotional processing. This reminiscing was ably assisted by time (wakes went on for three to four days) and that very potent abreactant, alcohol (to abreact: to assist in the process of emotional integration through recall). All this has disappeared along with the village, or is no longer available to the same degree. Increasing levels of isolation, alienation and loneliness are found in our sanitised, segregated and impersonal towns and cities. Counselling perhaps has also replaced the confessor or spiritual advisor. We now confess to our counsellor rather than to our priest or vicar. On top of this the dominant social discourse invites us to see 'normality' as being employed, happy, socially engaged etc. Many people find themselves falling well short of social norms, and this can reinforce their sense of isolation.

The rate of change in our present society is another important factor in the increased demand for counselling. In the past a person was often born into, lived and died in the same parish. Now we move to new parishes, provinces, countries, continents and set up home in many different places. We also live in a society with increasingly multifaceted choices available. Will we eat Cantonese or Mexican this evening? Health care is an area where the number and complexities of choices have increased greatly over the past 50 years. This is in part due to the success of new treatments. If we experience cardiac pain, for example, we may have a series of decisions to make: are we going to have cardiac angiography and, depending on the results of this test, cholesterol-lowering drugs or bypass surgery?

The increased complexity of choices has also been added to by our unwillingness to rely on traditional answers to current problems. Old certainties are giving way to uncertainty: should a couple stay together or apart and/or how many children will they decide to have if they decide to stay together, and when will they have them? This rate and complexity of change requires mechanisms to help us accommodate and manage these changes. Counselling is one such mechanism. Access to expert counselling, we now argue, is no small matter as often the choices in health care carry major importance for our lives and our health.

EDUCATIONAL/INFORMATIONAL COUNSELLING

Implicit in what we have been considering thus far is a particular form of counselling; counselling around change/choice which is about processing information. We apply this type of counselling continually in the health service; for example, an in-depth explanation of what a diagnosis of diabetes might mean in terms of lifestyle, drug treatment etc. will often require counselling. The discovery of a genetic marker for the genetically transmitted disease Huntington's Chorea (a form of premature dementia) means we can test for the presence of the disease. For those with the disease in their family, the decision to have the test requires in-depth pre- and post-test counselling so that the full ramifications of such a test and its results are properly understood. Obviously this understanding is crucial for a couple considering having children. It could be said that most health care choices nowadays, because of their complexity, require adequate counselling and information, so that individuals can make truly informed choices.

Doctors in particular are now expected to outline all the risks and benefits of treatments to patients and to provide for a safe non-directive environment where patients can reflect and make their own decisions. Such counselling/education is required so that patients can give fully informed consent. A woman who seeks tubal ligation needs to have the risk and possibility of post-operative pregnancy fully explained to her. Pre-test counselling for HIV needs to address the emotional, financial and insurance implications as well as the physical consequences of testing positive. The list of counselling situations in health care is endless. It is clear that doctors, nurses, psychologists and social workers require adequate counselling skills in order to keep patients informed and fully cognisant of their rights and choices. Failure to provide for such counselling can constitute, in its extreme form, negligence. This complexity has consequences for counsellors, where considerable skill is often required to help an individual decide on subtle and complex issues. For example, a counsellor may need to be educationally directive in giving advice about diet to a diabetic and in the next session to be non-directive with a couple deciding on family planning choices. These switches of role require subtlety and clarity on behalf of the counsellor. This type of counselling we might term educational/ informational counselling (type 1).

EMOTIONAL INTEGRATION COUNSELLING

A second type of counselling concerns itself more with emotional integration (type 2). This relates in broad terms to two areas. The first of these could be called expected life transitions such as birth, puberty, marriage, birth of children, graduation, promotion, loss of a job, retirement and death. All of these natural life transitions bring with them changes of role and identity which may carry emotional consequences. As referred to above, in traditional cultures these life transitions are marked by ceremonial and ritual which assist emotional integration. Some of these life transitions may be traumatic by their nature, e.g. loss of a job, or some may not, such as marriage.

Those in the health care field need to be aware of a person's failure to make such transitions successfully and, where there is difficulty, of the value of early intervention to prevent abnormal adjustment and/or psychological or psychiatric illness. Work to assist emotional integration may be required when a person has experienced trauma at the time of a transition. The work of John Bowlby (1973) and Elizabeth Kubler-Ross (1979) is of interest here. They have described the natural stages of emotional integration of traumatic events. These stages are:

1   Shock

2   Denial

3   Grieving

4   Bargaining

5   Acceptance

6   Work centred on others.

Failure to move through these stages within a reasonable time frame may require the intervention of counselling. In the death of a relative, for example, emotional ambivalence towards the dead person may block full grieving and emotional resolution of the person's death. Receiving a diagnosis of major illness may constitute such trauma. The patient who has been told that they have asthma, ulcerative colitis or perhaps even cancer may need considerable counselling. This counselling will need to address both informational/educational counselling (type 1) and the emotional impact of such a diagnosis (type 2). Failure to integrate the emotional impact of such a diagnosis can have a detrimental outcome on the course of the illness itself. Often this failure will manifest as non-compliance with medication, be that in medical or psychiatric illness.

Such failure to emotionally integrate a diagnosis is a common problem in psychiatry. Major psychiatric diagnoses often carry extra emotional impact, because the person may feel that society will now consider them to be a failure as a person, or may look on them as a second-class citizen. Failure to address these emotional issues in counselling may lead to denial of the illness, an inability on behalf of the patient to follow through properly with required treatment, and frequent relapse. This need for counselling may also apply to the families of patients who have been given a psychiatric diagnosis. The work of Julian Leff (1982) with patients who have been diagnosed with schizophrenia and their families has clearly shown that educational and counselling inputs can reduce the number of hospital admissions for such patients. Here the counselling task may be complex, with a need to educate families towards greater understanding of the illness and at the same time help them to find more appropriate ways of coping with problems that arise, as well as working on family attitudes towards patients. Families in which a member has been diagnosed to have schizophrenia, with the best of intentions, can tend to take on decision making for the identified family member or be overly sensitive to living skills difficulties, and thereby inadvertently block the person's development of self-reliance. Counselling work with such families has had measurable outcomes in reducing hospital admission.

We could further sub-type this second form of counselling. The focus is still emotional integration of trauma, but in the context of major trauma or a catastrophic event. There is a difference of degree between these sub-types. When an event is experienced as catastrophic, be it personal or group, there can be great difficulty in emotional integration. This appears to be due to the perceived life-threatening nature of such events. Rape and sexual abuse of children come under this category. In the modern health care setting, a staff member suffering a needle-stick injury may constitute such a traumatic event. Catastrophes can also occur to a group of people, as in the Zeebrugge ferry disaster or the Stardust fire. There now seems to be ample evidence that when such traumatic events occur and are perceived to be life-threatening, the person disassociates emotionally. Magee (1984) describes some attributes of the shock phase as follows: during such incidents a person will often describe how time appeared to slow down or stand still. They also report a greatly increased clarity of the sense faculties. It would appear as though there is an evolutionary advantage to being unaware of the emotional impact during the actual traumatic event itself, for example, the soldier who is oblivious to the bullet wound until after the battle. Thus the person makes the necessary behavioural actions needed to maximise their chances of survival without being hampered by the emotional reaction to such an event. In other words, the person gets stuck in the shock phase.

After such an event, the person may spontaneously integrate the emotional impact. This usually takes the form of a strong emotional reaction. However, the necessary emotional integration after the event does not always occur. In these instances the necessary integration can be greatly assisted by talking through the details of the event so that the emotional impact can be felt, experienced and integrated. In other words, early debriefing can help the individual move from the shock stage to emotional awareness of the impact of the event. There has been a move towards the high-profile provision of such services during times of catastrophe. However, there are indicators that follow-up counselling is often inadequate. An example of this is the Lockerbie air disaster, where high-profile counselling was provided in the initial stages. However, the fact that the townspeople still avoid the actual plane crash site suggests that many of the community have not fully processed the emotional impact of that event in their lives. However, where successful, this type of intervention prevents longer term psychological sequels such as phobias, post traumatic stress disorder, unresolved grief, secondary depression etc.

In general terms, hospitalisations for serious illness can often constitute trauma of the catastrophic variety for an individual. The lack of counselling within various health care settings is at times quite noticeable and often complained of by both patients and their families. It must be said that the nursing profession are often ahead in this area. The emphasis on caring in their training often helps them to be more alert and responsive to the emotional needs of their patients. The strong emphasis on technological training of doctors has militated against the medical profession being as aware as it should be of such issues. That is not to say that all faculties of medicine around the world do not teach adequate counselling skills to young doctors. However, at undergraduate level there is a clear lack of comprehensive training for doctors – as well as for psychologists, social workers, nurses etc. – of type 1 and type 2 counselling skills.

COUNSELLING/PSYCHOTHERAPY

It is now time to consider a third form of counselling. In a way we could say this is more psychotherapy than counselling. While psychotherapy is beyond the remit of this paper, it will for completeness be given some consideration here. There is often confusion about what constitutes counselling and what is psychotherapy. Psychotherapy looks at the deeper foundations within us which make us who we are, our fundamental being in the world. It is arguable whether counselling can be seen to be involved in this area. It can however be said that some of this area is addressed in counselling as it is difficult to engage a person deeply without coming in touch with this fundamental aspect of the person. Therefore, because counselling easily crosses into this territory it is necessary to give it some consideration here.

Undoubtedly the grandfather of modern western psychotherapy is Sigmund

Freud. He first published a paper on this area just over one hundred years ago, in 1894. Psychoanalysis emphasises the inner experience of the individual and unconscious material which manifests as symptoms and neurotic patterns of behaviour. In certain forms of psychoanalysis, this unconscious material is interpreted by the expert analyst, thereby assisting the individual to bring material which is implicit to conscious awareness. It considers that an individual may fail to grow and develop mentally and may fixate on early patterns of behaviour. These patterns are laid down as the infant negotiates various stages, such as the oral, anal, genital. For example, a person fixated at the anal stage may work with the world through a pattern of needing to control and might present with obsessive behaviours. This model dominated psychotherapy for the first thirty years of this century.

In what could be seen to be a reaction against a very strong focus on inner psychic events, a second form of psychotherapy emerged, based on Learning Theory. Pavlov had shown that we can learn physiological responses and behaviours depending on what we experience as rewarding. Behaviourists focus on the development of this learned or conditioned response. In other words we learn, at a very deep physiological level, a certain way of behaving by being rewarded, either physiologically or psychologically, for that behaviour. For example, we may avoid a feared situation and be rewarded physiologically, by a drop in our levels of anxiety and tension. Repeated learned avoidance of feared situations may then lead to a full-blown phobic avoidant neurotic pattern of behaviour.

These two first waves of psychotherapy have a number of things in common, perhaps the most pertinent to our discussion being that they both rely heavily on an expert who guides the person through the therapeutic endeavour. The expert knows best how to treat the person, and the person places themselves in the hands of the psychoanalyst or behaviour therapist.

The second half of the twentieth century saw a third wave of psychological interventions. This third wave has been dominated by the Humanistic, Constructivist, Existential and Systemic schools of psychotherapy. A description of these newer schools and any in-depth exploration of psychotherapy are beyond the remit of this paper. For a fuller exposition of the Constructivist position see Kenny (1988) or Gunne and O'Sullivan (1993). The Systemic perspective, which owes much to the pioneering work of Gregory Bateson (1985), and the Existentialist perspective have particularly influenced group psychotherapy practice (Yalom, 1980), and newer psychoanalytic approaches owe much to the work of Lacan (1968). Because the Humanistic School has had a considerable influence on counselling, it will be considered in some detail. The work of Carl Rogers (1951) in particular is almost synonymous with humanistic counselling. Rogers developed a humanistic counselling method which he termed 'Client-Centred Therapy', emphasising the innate wisdom of the person, whom he saw as possessing a natural ability to find his or her own way through life. He postulated that all the counsellor needed to provide was the right conditions for this natural process to unfold. The right conditions were provided through the proper quality of relationship between the counsellor and the client. The counsellor needed to bring certain attributes or attitudes to the relationship in order to provide a safe space where natural healing could occur. These qualities Rogers defined as unconditional positive regard, which emphasises the recognition of the basic goodness of the person and acceptance of the person as they are, unconditionally, and the ability to know accurately how another is experiencing the world and reflect this back to them. The third essential attribute defined by Rogers was congruence, or the counsellor's ability to resonate with his/her own inner feeling/thinking states and reflect these within the therapeutic relationship. In certain ways Rogers' theory is common sense. It puts the focus on the way the counsellor relates to the client and goes about providing a safe atmosphere for the person to explore and find their own way. This safety of the counselling process is the critical factor in allowing for the natural unfolding of the person's own process, the counsellor does not have to do anything *to* the client.

Using Rogers' logic the person is central: it is their process and it needs to be guided by them. The expert fades into the background and is just expected to provide a space in which the client (no longer the patient) can work. The provision of the safe atmosphere becomes the work of the counsellor. In this safe space the client's own concerns guide the process, the language is theirs, the pacing and the understanding. In fact, it can be argued that this third wave of client-centred therapy/counselling has never really quite reached the health care professions and that we still tend to emphasise very much the expert stance. This is true in psychiatry as well as in the rest of medicine and often leads to a sense of alienation. This alienation is increased when highly technical interventions are used.

Rogers claimed that the ability to relate unconditionally, emphatically and congruently could be taught to individuals and he spent many years, in a number of universities in the USA, researching his method and his ability to train counsellors in it. The Rogerian approach can be seen to have ready application to what we have been discussing so far. Such an approach helps us at the informational level (type 1), where the client's autonomy is respected and a non-directive approach is emphasised. We can equally well see it is helpful for an individual who is in the process of emotional integration of life transitions and traumas (type 2).

However, the implications of Rogers' approach have a further consequence. Given this safe atmosphere and space, an individual may not just process information and/or unfold recent trauma and difficulty but may feel safe enough to begin to explore deeper trauma and failures of adaptation and integration of the personality present from the time of adolescence or earlier. This ability to access characterological maladaptive patterns brings Rogers' work into areas covered by Psychoanalysis and Behaviourism (type 3 counselling/psychotherapy). These types of psychotherapy then attempt to intervene at the level of the underlying personality using their theoretical stance. Humanistic counselling psychotherapy would not address these developmental areas specifically but rather would claim that unresolved conflicts emerge as the client feels safe enough to allow them to surface and strong enough to deal with them.

Attempts at characterological change carry with them some degree of controversy and debate. A question often asked is, should health care services be charged with the remit of funding techniques that attempt to change personality which relates to the growth of the person during their childhood and adolescence? Is the cost of such explorations strictly beyond the remit of health care provision? A further question, of effectiveness of such methods, will be discussed in a later section.

In summary, we can define three types of counselling intervention: informational/educational, emotional processing, and some addressing of more deeply ingrained patterns or ways of being in the world. Each type can be used alone or in combinations of two or three to offer support and assistance to patients. Counselling itself can be used alone or in conjunction with other treatment modalities. Increasingly in health care settings, treatment involves multimodal approaches. Counselling is often a crucial part of treatment packages, for example as quoted above with schizophrenia, the effectiveness of counselling offered alongside methadone maintenance for long term opiate dependent intravenous drug users (McLellan *et al.* 1993), or in relapse prevention after alcohol or opiate detoxification. These research papers all describe counselling as a critical component of multidisciplinary treatment packages with the addition of counselling improving outcomes, in terms of health gain.

Before moving on we need perhaps to look at a further dimension to counselling. In ten to twenty years we may look back and say we are currently in the fourth wave of counselling/psychotherapy growth. This has seen the introduction of the spiritual dimension into counselling/psychotherapy. This is a highly controversial development. The argument goes something like this: medicine in general has introduced increasing awareness of psychological and sociological factors, alongside the biological, as both predisposing factors, precipitating and perpetuating causes of disease, so why not the spiritual? In the USA in particular and to some extent in Europe there is a growing interest in this area. In its simplest and least esoteric form this dimension has been characterised by the concept of self-actualisation. Abraham Maslow along with Rogers introduced the concept of hierarchy of needs. These begin with the most simple and basic such as the need for shelter, food and clothing. Once these needs have been met more complex ones arrive at the top of our agenda, such as a need to form relationships, to belong, etc. Finally, if we satisfy all of our more basic needs we come to a point where we need to fulfil our full potential; this actualisation carries with it even notions of transcending ourselves.

Within the scope of fulfilling our potential, some would argue that we need to address the spiritual dimension of being human. This area has been off limits for counselling/psychotherapy for most of this century. Scientists have declared the spiritual dimension unmeasurable and thereby beyond the remit of science. On the other hand it can be argued that without this dimension we are leaving out a significant proportion of the human beingness, of who we are. Is, for example, the growth of addictions within our culture an attempt to fill the spiritual void in our lives? Can we call ourselves fully human without addressing our need to care for others and unfold our compassion? (Akong, 1994). Do these failures of compassionate expression affect our physical health? Is the spiritual dimension beyond science in being unmeasurable? A comprehensive coverage of this topic is beyond the scope of this chapter. It can be safely assumed that this type of intervention is at present outside the domain of health-funded therapy. However, it may be the cutting edge of newer developments in the field.

EFFECTIVENESS AND RESOURCES

Thus far we have been examining the different forms of counselling/ psychotherapy and the reasons for the increased demand for such interventions. The counterbalance to this increased demand is increasing competition for limited resources within health care budgets. More and more treatments are becoming available for different conditions. This brings us to the question of how effective psychotherapies and deeper counselling are at bringing about deeper personality change. The debate on their effectiveness has raged for over forty years – and research in the area is notoriously difficult.

In 1952 Eysenck claimed that neurotic patients on waiting lists did as well as those in psychotherapy (Eysenck, 1952). In 1982 the American Psychiatric Association Commission on the Psychotherapies, in a review of psychotherapy research, concluded that psychotherapy and counselling provide for real measurable change. This was based on research which had shown that change was non-specific and no differences in effect could be seen when comparing generic counselling and differing psychotherapeutic approaches (Smith and Glass, 1977). This research seemed to damn all counselling and psychotherapy with faint praise. Margison, reviewing psychotherapy research in 1989, concluded that there are many confounding difficulties, such as defining treatments and operationalising them in terms of research outcome, and similar difficulties around control groups and the provision of adequate placebos, as well as difficulties around choices of measures. However, despite all these problems, Margison concluded that the greatest difficulty in this area has been 'the unfortunate polarisation across a classic versus a romantic dimension which has blocked psychotherapy research much more effectively than any problems inherent in psychotherapy research design'. He suggests that 'a way through is for clinicians to see research as being clinically relevant and an accepted part of their own practice'.

It is legitimate for health managers to question the funding of prolonged treatment packages, and to seek valid and reliable research data to guide funding decisions (*Shaping a Healthier Future,* 1994). A leader in this field has been cognitive therapy (Beck, 1991), where controlled trials have shown this intervention to be highly effective in clinical depression. Despite this, the health care manager is still likely to fund quicker and relatively less expensive antidepressant chemotherapy over a cognitive approach. The tide however may soon turn. If cognitive therapy can be shown to reduce significantly the recurrence of depression, then the cost ratio sums may work out in psychotherapy's favour. This research is being undertaken. Some further ways forward may include the use of specific techniques for specific types of illness and character traits. For example, the avoidant/phobic patient may do best with behavioural approaches, while the depressed patient may benefit most from cognitive therapy. Given the potential benefits of such approaches and of their high cost, it is critical that psychotherapists and counsellors who wish to work in the area of deeper characterological change address these research issues. Well controlled randomised trials need to be conducted so that funding can be based on proven efficiency and effectiveness.

We need also to look at informational/educational counselling (type 1 counselling) and the effectiveness of this type of intervention. In a certain sense we can answer the question rather easily, for type 1, and simply say that it is medicolegally required that health care professionals inform people properly of their conditions and choices of treatment. It seems therefore that we need this type of counselling. Other work, such as that of Leff referred to earlier, also indicates the benefit of type 1 counselling. The effectiveness of emotional interpretation of information/trauma (type 2) is a somewhat different matter; this usually requires a number of sessions and often involves type 1 informational work as well. It would appear that in relatively straightforward work around life transitions, emotional integration can be assisted by counselling and thereby more serious psychological/psychiatric sequels can be prevented (Waldron, 1984). More controversy surrounds counselling type 2 b where the focus is a catastrophe or severe immediate trauma out of the ordinary expected experience. The counselling technique which has dominated this area was first called 'critical incident stress debriefing' (CISD), which was later changed to 'psychological debriefing' (PD). A report in 1994 concluded that PD was unlikely to influence the outcome of such events as much as the acute stress reaction, previous history of trauma, personality, past psychiatric history, and the adequacy of social supports (Bisson and Deahl, 1994). However, other studies have been more hopeful. A more comprehensive package offered to soldiers traumatised in the Gulf War – a 12-day structured inpatient course of highly focused group psychotherapy including type 1 educational counselling, discussion, problem solving, recall of personal trauma experiences and family reintegration, followed by crisis line support from counsellors and day-case follow up over a one-year period – was found to significantly reduce morbidity (Busuttil *et al.* 1995). The study of these Gulf War veterans, however, was on a small number and was not a controlled trial.

Other techniques have had favourable results in post traumatic stress disorder (PTSD). Particular mention should be made of eye movement desensitisation and reprocessing (EMDR). In a number of controlled trials, this brief intervention technique has been shown to be superior to a variety of alternatives for PTSD (MacCulloch and Feldman, 1996). The research into types 1 & 2 counselling suggests that, when done properly by professionally trained counsellors/psychotherapists, with proper follow-through, this type of counselling does reduce the likelihood of psychological (e.g. prolonged unresolved grief) and psychiatric (e.g. post bereavement depression, post traumatic stress disorder) sequel. But more controlled trials do need to be completed in this area. This is not to say that all require this form of intervention; as we have seen, many people can process emotionally with the help of conventional rituals and ceremonies. Nor should all have equal quantities/quality of intervention – some will need more or less depending on the trauma and the individual. However, it is clear that it is at least good prevention to offer this type of intervention to patients who fail to emotionally integrate severe trauma and where there are signs of psychological decompensation. What is becoming increasingly clear is that not all techniques work equally well. Counsellors need very detailed and comprehensive skills training based on the best available research at hand. This research itself must be critically evaluated. It is no longer possible to fund all options. We need to prioritise so that we can offer the most effective methods to those in need. If it were cardiac surgery we would expect this. When it comes to our minds, why should we settle for less?

ACCREDITATION AND TRAINING

How are we to ensure such standards are met? In other disciplines this is left to the universities. They set standards of training which provide the basis for professional practice. Here in Ireland we have developed university courses with diplomas and certificates and degrees in counselling. University College and Trinity College in Dublin, as well as Cork University and the University of Ulster, have certificate and degree courses in psychology counselling. Others such as Maynooth have extra-mural counselling courses. University College Dublin and Queen's University, Belfast have masters' degrees in psychotherapy for those from medical, psychological and sociological backgrounds. This plethora of courses attests to the urgent need to set up Faculties of Counselling and Psychotherapy. A formal request to set up such a Faculty or Faculties needs to be made to the Departments of Health and Education. This request is being made on the Department of Health's fiftieth birthday. Perhaps a birthday is a good time to ask for something!

The wealth of research alone in this area is difficult to track. There is a need to oversee the specialised continued education and training now required to stay abreast of the field. Many claim that counselling and psychotherapy have failed to prove efficacy and have generally not been answerable to the larger body politic. This accusation has some truth, with some notable exceptions, including the work of professionals in our country. On the other hand counselling and psychotherapy are very young sciences and are arguably the most complex – what, after all, is more complex than the human being? What is beginning to emerge slowly is that the art of psychologically facilitating healthy transitions in life, the science of providing proper education/ information as well as the safe space in which to process it, and the deep science of changing ingrained patterns of behaviour present since childhood which determine our ways of being with others, are not easy skills to learn. Nor are necessarily complex techniques the best approaches. Often people respond best to simple interventions. We need to demystify counselling and empower people. However, windows are opening. We are beginning to learn how to do certain small things well. We need a properly appointed faculty or faculties to co-ordinate the surging tide of new data into meaningful clinical methods and in turn to contribute to this research. How to do good quantative and qualitative research in counselling and psychotherapy is a question being asked by many clinicians and teachers in Ireland.

Accreditation and training of counsellors is another highly topical issue. In this regard, the European dimension has played a major role in recent developments in Ireland. The challenge of mutual recognition of psychotherapy training has spurred the counselling and psychotherapy professions to formalise training and accreditation standards in Ireland. Recently, in many European countries as well as Ireland, non-statutory Registers of Psychotherapists have been established. The Irish Council for Psychotherapy has just published the first such register of accredited psychotherapists in Ireland (1997). Counsellors too have formed the Irish Association of Counselling and Therapy and the Irish Association of Alcohol and Addiction Counsellors. All of these specify basic minimum standards of training and standards are going up all the time.

Recently a pan-European body has been formed with the aim of establishing psychotherapy as an independent profession, the European Association of Psychotherapists. This Association in turn is working to accredit psychotherapists who reach a certain standard with a European Certificate of Psychotherapy. In order to receive a certificate a person will have to show proof of undergraduate training in a health care field such as sociology, psychology, medicine or nursing where the basic human sciences will have been covered. This will be followed by four years of specialist training. These four years will cover theories of personality developmental, psychology and basic psychotherapy approaches, as well as clinical skills training. Finally those certifying will need to specialise in recognised and researched forms of counselling and psychotherapy, a total of seven years' training in all. Such a specialised training needs to be under one roof. Already in some European universities we are seeing the appointment of professors of counselling and psychotherapy. We urgently need to follow suit so that we can have the very best psychological care available for ourselves and for our children.

However, these developments in specialised training for counsellors do not dispense with an urgent and ongoing need to provide properly systematised counselling training for health care professionals such as nurses, psychologists, social workers and doctors. People skills are vital to these disciplines. There is some evidence of increasing awareness, as some of the professional training courses have begun to include at least small modules on counselling. The IMO has recently set up an expert group to review counselling training for general practitioners. Psychiatry too has begun to look in this direction – note for example the work of John Barker, Professor of Psychiatric Nursing at the University of Newcastle (Barker, 1995). He has emphasised that psychiatry needs to move to a client-centred approach if it is to retain patients. Many psychiatric patients are seeking counselling in the private sector because of the continued adoption of an expert authoritarian stance by both psychiatric nurses and psychiatrists. Barker has insisted that there is a need to relate more with the actual experience of the patient, to bring a client-centred approach to patients experiencing psychiatric illness. Professor of Psychiatry Julian Leff has also added considerably to our understanding of how skilful counselling techniques can help in the treatment of schizophrenia. In very elegant research work, he has shown that families who live with a person diagnosed as schizophrenic can learn to cope more successfully with effects of the illness. This safe environment can reduce relapse rates and the need for high dose medication. Dr. Edward Podvoll has shown similar results by providing client-centred sane environments for patients suffering from psychotic illnesses (Podvoll, 1990). Supportive counselling added to pharmacotherapy has been shown to be effective in the treatment of addictions (McLellan *et al.*, 1993) and in other psychiatric disorders (Leff, 1982). As we have seen, without it patients often do poorly on medication alone.

Counselling and psychotherapy as we have known them are in the process of rapid change. The standards expected are very high. Side effects, such as false memory syndrome, have increasingly been recognised. Costs are a constraining factor as are skills and proper training as well as access to the most authoritative research. Despite the difficulties there is a strong demand for client-centred approaches. What then is the deep appeal of these methods? To answer this question we need to look at the philosophical roots of this approach. The humanistic and existentialist philosophical traditions of the late nineteenth and early twentieth centuries have attempted to put human meaning and experience back in the centre of our existence. These philosophies are phenomenological in that they put our experience as humans as the centre ground of who we are. It would appear as though these philosophies have grown out of the realisation that the human race has had to come to terms with the fact that the earth is not the centre of the solar system, nor is our solar system the centre of our galaxy, nor is our galaxy the centre of the universe. At the same time, scientific explorations of natural science have called into question the uniqueness of the human condition in terms of evolutionary theory, animal instinctual drives and the way behaviour can be shaped. Similarly the human sciences of medicine, sociology and psychology continually break down (analyse) the human being into smaller and smaller sub-parts (i.e. we are a collection of atoms, but do even atoms exist?) which tends to add to the sense of meaninglessness to our lives.

The phenomenological approach of the humanistic and existential philosophies, by emphasising our experience of the world, have put the experience of being human back at the centre of the universe. In other words our given human experience becomes central and the part of us that is unique.

According to these traditions meaning can only come from within ourselves, and we can only start from where we find ourselves. We find ourselves existing and experiencing. The human sciences of medicine, psychology, sociology and psychiatry, according to this analysis, have failed to take adequate account of this third wave and have rather focused on the biological, cognitive and social components of our experience. In other words, focused on the parts that we are made of. This is what many patients complain of when they are confronted by modern western medicine. They speak of being treated as if they are on a conveyor belt, talked to as if only their diseased organ is of interest, talked down to, around and dismissed. What modern western medicine is only gradually becoming aware of is that it is only by taking cognisance of the human and very personal experience of being ill, and putting this personal experience in the context of the person's own life, that we can become truly human in our approach, to our patients and clients.

FUTURE NEEDS

Where to for the future? Counselling appears to be here to stay. Whatever about the values of various counselling techniques as treatment – and much more work needs to be done to ascertain the best technique for the circumstances presented – there is a need for a broad-based counselling approach to patients. This approach, which is highly respecting of their physical, psychological, sociological and spiritual integrity, is all about relationships and the way health care professionals relate to the people they treat. We need counselling which is professional, yet inexpensive and available when needed, just like primary education. Specific techniques need to be vigorously researched and counsellors systematically trained in their use. Like the introduction of primary education in the last century, basic counselling as a right should be available to all, in all health care settings, i.e. the right to be a human being and have someone talk to us, explaining what is going on to us, consulting us, getting our views and opinions, informing us and getting our truly informed and clear consent. The ability to educate and to listen to our patients is critically important to help them process information and their emotional reactions to that information. Similarly, skilled counselling can help people to cope better with traumas or change. Providing good quality counselling at the right time to people who need it makes good psychological sense as well as probably being very good preventative medicine. At the same time we need to formalise training standards and accreditation procedures within the universities and professional associations.

All health care disciplines need basic training in the counselling skills of empathic listening and congruent relationships and we definitely need to honour, respect and accept our patients and clients as the human beings they are. The relationships we form with our patients/clients are of primary importance. Many will have heard senior clinicians emphasise listening to the history of the patient or to the mother of a child when trying to diagnose an illness. All of this comes back to a very old skill, bedside manner. We also need trained specialist counsellors to work with more complex, informational and emotional processing, for example pre-and post-testing counselling for serious illness such as HIV or genetically transmitted illnesses and for those suffering symptoms of post traumatic stress. These counsellors should not be an expert elite but rather integrated into health care teams. The question of more in-depth therapeutic approaches which focus on in-depth characterological change awaits further research and validation, although there is evidence of some benefit from specific methods for specific psychological/psychiatric illnesses.

Above all we need to build into our biological, psychological and sociological models a view of the human being as multi-dimensional, including perhaps even the spiritual. Are we fully addressing a total human being when we leave this dimension out? 'Believing is seeing' according to Maturan (Maturan and Varela, 1988). With these newer humanistic models of the human being perhaps we can 'see' the person in front of us. For the present we need to do simple things well rather than overreach ourselves and discredit what is essential. Counselling is essential, because in health care we are after all dealing with human beings, who have feelings and need to plan for the future and to put their lives in a meaningful context. Failure to provide for these basic human needs, because we are too busy with the latest technology or research refinements, is to dishonour, disempower and above all to dehumanise our patients/clients and ourselves.

CHAPTER 12

Medico-Legal and Ethical Issues

Denis A. Cusack

Major concern with medico-legal and medico-ethical issues was once confined to the lofty thinkers of medicine, law and philosophy. The majority of healthcare practitioners got on with the task of caring for their patients to the best of their abilities without having to give undue thought to the legal and ethical implications of their practice. But this is no longer so and medical law and ethics now impinge on healthcare practice on a daily basis. Whether the enormous changes in the social, political and scientific areas of medicine have effected change in fields of medical law and medical ethics in the past fifty years or not is a matter for debate in the overall context of healthcare delivery.

There is a recognition of the role now played by legal medicine in healthcare. Unfortunately in many people's minds the role of medical law and ethics is perceived as negative and divisive and illustrated by the increase in litigation for professional negligence, the debates about abortion or the withdrawal of food and hydration in patients in the persistent vegetative state.

Legal medicine encompasses medical law, medical ethics, clinical forensic medicine, thanatology (study of death), forensic pathology, toxicology and poisoning and healthcare legislation. This essay addresses the first two of these divisions of the speciality.

The relationship between medical law and ethics has been and should be close. Law is the concretisation of the mores of society and should reflect the ethical principles of that society. However, in the sphere of healthcare it must now be realised that on occasion there is a divergence between medical law and ethics. Perhaps this is not surprising, since judges interpret law whereas healthcare professionals, as their name implies, provide healthcare for their patients. The roles of judges and healthcarers are different by their very nature.

There is an increasing awareness of medico-legal and medico-ethical matters by both healthcare professionals and by patients. Legal medicine, or at least parts of it, is now included in the education of many healthcare professionals at both undergraduate and postgraduate levels and as part of continuing professional development. Medical law is a subject included in the curricula of an increasing number of law schools. Why is there this interest and need? Is it driven merely by the increase in the number of actions taken by patients against healthcare institutions and carers? Or is it a recognition of the need to improve medico-legal and related skills in order to deliver a better healthcare system to the patient?

Medical law and ethics have a legally derived major input from statutory bodies such as the Medical Council and An Bord Altranais[1] as well as from the non-statutory professional bodies such as the Irish Society of Chartered Physiotherapists. These bodies provide codes of conduct for their respective professions. The Department of Health, on behalf of the government of the people, obviously also plays a major role through formulating general healthcare policy. Increasingly in the future patient groups and consumer groups will be heard more strongly in the areas of patient rights, patient choice and patient autonomy. The emergence of the fledgling Irish Patients Association in 1996 is to be welcomed.

How then have medical law and ethics evolved since 1947? There are many issues in both of these areas which reflect the changes in healthcare practice in the past few decades and which point the way to the future.

PATIENT AUTONOMY AND CONSENT

Perhaps the most fundamental change has been in the status of the patient. The ways in which patients view themselves and how they are viewed by healthcare professionals have altered. We are moving from a paternalistic approach to patient healthcare to one which increasingly has to recognise the emergence of patient autonomy. Prior to the 1980s, patient autonomy was not a major issue in Ireland. Legal cases concerning patient consent reflected this. The cases of Bolam[2] and Sidaway[3] in England left decision making for patients quite firmly in the hands of the medical profession with some token input from the patient. However, the 1992 case of Walsh[4] set out the disclosure of risks which must be given for consent to elective or non-essential procedures in Ireland and required a fuller disclosure from healthcarers than had been the practice heretofore. The Farrell[5] case looked back to the more paternalistic approach. Taken together, these two cases have left Irish medical law on consent in a state of confusion (Donnelly, 1996) but there can be little doubt that the 'doctor knows best and don't worry yourself' approach is dead. The patient's right to know is now firmly established. Patients of the 1990s must be sufficiently informed and sufficiently free to consent to medical intervention (Medical Council, 1994).

PATIENT REFUSAL AND ADVANCE DIRECTIVES

One aspect of patient autonomy which has been receiving much attention relates to the right of a patient to refuse treatment even when the consequences of such refusal may threaten the health or life of the patient. If the patient has the required legal capacity and the refusal is an informed one and made voluntarily, then such a refusal is valid and recognised in law.

The advance directive or 'living will' is also an expression of patient autonomy. The directive sets out the wishes of the patient in relation to healthcare decisions in anticipation of a particular circumstance arising which would render the patient incapable of making such decisions (Law Commission, 1995). The legal standing of such a document is not entirely clear in the Irish jurisdiction although the right of a patient to refuse treatment itself is beyond doubt. The problem arises in enforcing such advance directives if the medical and nursing staff do not believe that they accord with the ethical principles of patient care (BMA, 1995).

Decision making on behalf of the incompetent patient is an even more difficult topic. Who can properly exercise that right and what are the safeguards for the patient? The Powers of Attorney Act 1996 allows a person to confer on another person the authority to make decisions when the donor of the power is becoming mentally incapable. However, the legislation did not include provision for decisions on healthcare matters. This is an area yet to be addressed.

MENTAL HEALTH LAW

The Mental Treatment Act, 1945 still governs the prevention and treatment of mental disorders and the care of persons suffering from such disorders. Yet has not forensic psychiatry progressed since that time? How much more enlightened is our understanding of mental disease in the 1990s?

The duration of detention of involuntary patients under the Act has decreased very significantly since the 1950s to the extent that 83-86% of such patients were discharged within three months in the period 1991-1993 (Irish Health Research Board, 1993). The 1995 Government White Paper proposed a more restrictive definition of mental disorder to include mental illness, significant mental handicap and severe dementia but expressly excluded personality disorder and social deviance (paras 2.8-2.17). It also proposed that alcohol and drug addiction be excluded from the definition (para 2.20). These proposed legal changes reflect an improved medical and social understanding of these conditions.

The proposed strengthening of safeguards for the involuntary patient are more in line with the modern requirements of the European Convention on Human Rights, the United Nation Principles and the Council of Europe recommendation for the legal protection of this group of patients. The proposed Mental Health Review Board (paras 5.11-5.22) with an appeal mechanism, the requirements for consent and a second opinion for psychosurgery and the appointment of a Commissioner of Mental Health (paras 10.5-10.8) for the protection of patients all reflect a changing attitude to persons with mental illness and their rights under the law. The proposal for adult care orders (paras 8.6-8.9) also reflects a growing awareness of a desire to protect the vulnerable adult in a caring society. Concerns have been expressed in relation to a number of aspects of the proposed legislation, including the practicality of a senior psychiatrist reviewing a patient prior to involuntary admission, and the role of the District Court in the process (Webb, 1995; Spellman, 1995).

CHILDCARE LEGISLATION AND CHILD ABUSE

Another vulnerable section of society are our children. Medical law and ethics have been no less active in this sphere. The social changes in child care, and in particular in relation to residential care, adoption and the rights of children, are reflected in the very public debate on child welfare and well-being. The Child Care Act 1991, which updated the law in relation to the care of children previously governed by the Children Act 1908, has now been fully implemented. It seeks to protect children who have been assaulted, ill-treated, neglected or sexually abused or who are at risk. It also provides for inspection and supervision of pre-school services and for registration and inspection of residential centres for children. The number of reported incidences of child abuse has risen dramatically from 405 in 1982 to 6,415 in 1995[6]. The Child Abuse Guidelines of 1987 have been amended by a 1995[7] document in relation to the circumstances in which the health boards and the Gardai notify suspected cases of child abuse to each other. The 1993 Kilkenny Incest Investigation and the 1996 Report of the Irish Catholic Bishops Advisory Committee are further proof of the enormous changes in attitude to and thinking about what had been previously a taboo subject.

The government at the end of 1996 decided not to introduce mandatory reporting of child abuse following submissions from over two hundred sources, including most professional healthcare and childcare organisations, and following a plenary meeting on the topic – although this will be reviewed at the end of the decade (*Putting Children First,* 1996, 1997). The legal and ethical roles of healthcarers and other professionals in reducing the incidence of child abuse will be a matter of major interest for many years to come.

PROFESSIONAL NEGLIGENCE

The increase in incidence of negligence claims by patients against hospitals, doctors, nurses and healthcare professionals in general is often cited as the most disturbing development in the heretofore trusting carer-patient relationship. Fifty years ago a negligence action by a patient against a doctor, nurse or hospital was a rarity.

Today in Ireland we have the dubious distinction of having the highest litigation rate in Europe and are second only to the United States in this activity. A doctor in Ireland is about four times more likely to be sued than his counterpart in Britain and eleven times more likely to be sued than a doctor in Hong Kong. Settlements and awards are approximately two to three times greater than those in Britain. There is a perceived rise in the practice of defensive medicine and a real escalation in the cost of indemnity subscriptions for doctors and insurance premia for hospitals on behalf of their institutions and their healthcare employees. It is anticipated that the taxpayer will pay in the region of £25 million pounds for doctors' malpractice indemnity in 1997. In 1952 the indemnity subscription for a doctor was £1, in 1978 it was £40, in 1988 the figure was £1,100 and in 1997 the individual medical practitioner in obstetrics faces a subscription of £35,000. In a recent publication on medical negligence, the author states that '[I]t is . . . simply wrong to suggest that patients, or lawyers, are responsible in any way for this admitted crisis . . .' (White, 1996). But who, or what, is responsible?

The cost to all involved in healthcare, both providers and those in receipt, goes beyond mere money. The psychological cost of the breakdown of the trusting relationship and its projection into the adversarial field of the courts is real and underestimated.

In this respect, the change from minimal litigation to an explosion of claims over the past decades may be seen as a very negative development. But it should also be viewed as a challenge to government and healthcare providers to identify the underlying problems and to look for solutions. The right of the injured patient to seek compensation for injuries brought about by poor standards of care must be defended as vigorously as the good name and reputation of the healthcarer who has carried out duties to the proper and competent standard. The introduction of alternative systems to adversarial litigation has been mooted. These include mediation and arbitration of disputes between patient and carers, the establishment of pre-trial screening tribunals to filter out non-meritorious claims, a no-fault compensation system for injuries such as the birth hypoxia brain-damaged baby, the introduction of structured settlements and the capping of personal injury awards (Law Reform Commission, 1997). Any reform must be set in the context of quality of service and accountability and must include the participation of all healthcare professionals, including healthcare management, and the emerging patient interest groups.

HEALTHCARE RISK MANAGEMENT AND STANDARDS OF PRACTICE

No single approach will resolve the litigation crisis. However, the recent recognition of healthcare risk management as part of the answer to the problem is also a concrete response by healthcarers and healthcare institutions to the need for delivery of quality service to the public. The process is one whereby risks to the patient are identified and anticipated and measures put in place to eliminate or minimise those risks (Cusack, 1994). The process also deals with the management through proper complaints procedures of potential claims in situations where accidents have already occurred. This is an example of a proactive approach to the inevitable problems which must arise in delivery of a complex healthcare service. It is unfortunate that it has taken an explosion in medical litigation to bring about this attitude.

In the blood transfusion scandal, originating in 1976 but still being acted out in 1997, professional healthcare standards have been under severe scrutiny and have been found wanting[8]. It is a profound irony that blood and blood products produced to improve the health of so many patients on a scale hardly imaginable in the 1940s have now injured 1,600 men, women and children on an equally unimaginable scale (Cusack, 1996). There must never be a recurrence.

PATIENT CONFIDENTIALITY AND MEDICAL RECORDS

'Whatever, in connection with my professional practice or not in connection with it, I see or hear in the life of men which ought not to be spoken of abroad, I will not divulge, as reckoning that all such should be kept secret'. This translated quotation from the Hippocratic Oath dates far beyond the last five decades but is as relevant today as ever. Certain aspects of confidentiality have been given modern twists by improved communications, computer technology and the voracious appetite of the hungry news media. Never has it been more important for healthcarers to safeguard clinical information of their patients and only to release information in accordance with legal and ethical guidelines

(O'Neill, 1995). The increasing complexity of decisions to be made by healthcarers and the conflict of duties which can arise is illustrated by the Medical Council's inquiry in a recent case where the duty of confidentiality owed by a doctor to patients and affected third parties was confirmed to extend beyond the third party's death (O'Toole, 1997). With increasing technology, personal databasing by government departments and the use of mobile telephones, faxes, e-mail and medical computer databases, vigilance and security will become even more important in the future[9].

At present only computer-held personal data are covered by legislation under the Data Protection Act 1988. It is inevitable that written and typewritten clinical notes will also be covered by specific legislation in the future which will safeguard the rights of the patient and will give a statutory right to the patient to access those records, a right which does not exist at the present time.

HEALTHCARERS AND PATIENTS WITH INFECTIOUS DISEASES

In the 1940s and 1950s the prevalence of tuberculosis in Irish society was a recognised risk for healthcarers involved in the diagnosis and treatment of infected patients. Exposure to the risk of infection was accepted by healthcarers and in the words of the Medical Council 'is a time-honoured tradition of the medical profession'[10]. Doctors and nurses were infected and some died as a result. In the 1990s concern has been expressed that patients may become infected by healthcarers who carry communicable diseases such as hepatitis B, hepatitis C and HIV. Should patients have a legal and enforceable right to be informed if their carer is HIV positive? What are the rights of the healthcarers who become infected through their employment?

Screening of healthcarers for these diseases and restricted access by infectious carers to exposure-prone techniques has been called for. Yet is it desirable that employing authorities and professional organisations should lay down rigid guidelines in relation to screening? The scientific basis for the effectiveness of this remains to be proved conclusively and the introduction of mandatory screening is a step to be taken only after serious consideration of the effectiveness and consequences of such a programme[11]. The answer to this may indeed be 'mutual trust based on an open exchange of information' (para 45.03), but is this sufficient? Put more strongly, there is an ethical and legal onus on both healthcarers and patients not to expose any other person knowingly or through recklessness to infection with a health-threatening or life-threatening infection. Personal responsibility is a facet of modern society which requires emphasis in law and ethics.

'RIGHT TO DIE'

This inexact term can have a number of meanings for different people. Is it about the right to die, or the right to be allowed to die, or the right to choose to die with dignity, or about the right to choose to be killed? Proponents and opponents of the 'right to die' have both been guilty of disingenuous inexactitude in the use of the term. Must the right not also encompass the right to life, and duties to others and to society generally to preserve life, whilst at the same time recognising the right of the individual to self-determination?

Perhaps the case of the patient known as The Ward has come to symbolise the difficulties of modern medicine and healthcare provision as no other case could have. The patient was deemed to be in a 'near persistent vegetative state' following anoxic brain damage subsequent to three cardiac arrests during a minor gynaecological procedure. On the issue of withdrawal of nutrition and hydration, medical law and medical ethics in Ireland truly diverged. The Supreme Court upheld the order of the High Court consenting to the withdrawal of what it deemed to be medical treatment. The Medical Council disagreed and stated that 'access to nutrition and hydration is one of the basic needs of human beings. This remains so even when, from time to time, this need can only be fulfilled by means of long established methods such as . . . gastrostomy tube feeding.' An Bord Altranais reaffirmed the need to provide nutrition and hydration for the patient[12].

It is now clear in the 1990s that what is lawful in accordance with judicial decision and what is ethical in accordance with medical and nursing guidelines are no longer automatically synonymous and medical opinion does not always agree with judicial decisions on healthcare issues (O'Brien, 1995). The Ward case illustrates the increasing complexity of the dilemmas thrown up by modern medical care. The issues raised by the case and to be addressed further include those of consent, patient autonomy, sacredness of life, categorisation of cognitive and brainstem functions, different levels of care and treatment (basic, nursing and medical) and decision making on behalf of incompetent patients.

Guidance and leadership on the many complex medical, ethical and legal dilemmas raised by the case are lacking. There is an urgent need for a review of the criteria for definition of persistent vegetative state and for the provision of medical care and treatment in chronic and terminal diseases within the context of proper respect for the sanctity of human life. The British Medical Association has issued guidelines for practitioners in the British jurisdiction[13]. There is no less a need for the Irish situation.

PHYSICIAN-ASSISTED SUICIDE

Active euthanasia and physician-assisted suicide, involving the intentional killing of a patient, are issues which are receiving increasing attention worldwide. The Supreme Court of the United States recently heard legal and medical submissions in two appeal cases involving patients seeking physician-assisted suicide. In both cases the court upheld the criminal laws which would have prevented such manner of suicide[14]. In Australia the Northern Territory passed legislation, the Rights of the Terminally Ill Act, which legalised physician-assisted suicide, although the legislation was subsequently overturned at federal level. Active euthanasia in the Netherlands remains a criminal offence but a doctor assisting a patient to commit suicide may be granted immunity from prosecution if certain pre-conditions or cumulative requirements originally set down by the Royal Dutch Medical Association are met. These include a voluntary and durable request to die by the patient which is well-informed and well-considered; there must be intolerable and hopeless suffering, no acceptable alternative left and consultation with a second physician. In Ireland the position on active euthanasia is clear: it is illegal and constitutes professional misconduct.

MEDICAL FUTILITY

The withdrawal of medical interventions which are deemed futile is in keeping with the ethical and legal principles of patient care. It is a recognition of patient autonomy and of the principles of patient beneficence and non-maleficence. The main determination to be made is which interventions are futile and which are not. With increasing medical technology this has become an everyday issue for intensive care nurses and doctors in the 1990s and one which is likely to become more complex in the future (Phelan and Kinirons, 1996; Tomkin and Hanafin, 1995).

RIGHT TO LIFE OF THE UNBORN

The insertion into the Constitution by referendum of the people in 1983 of an amendment to protect the life of the unborn had an unexpected if not wholly unforeseen outcome in the judgment of the X Case in 1992 when the Supreme Court ruled that '. . . if it is established as a matter of probability that there is a real and substantial risk to the life, as distinct from the health, of the mother, which can only be avoided by the termination of her pregnancy, such termination is permissible, having regard to the true interpretation of Article 40, s.3, sub-s. 3 of the Constitution'[15].

Criminal abortions were carried out in Ireland of the 1940s and 1950s. The prosecution of Nurse Mary Anne Cadden in 1956 was one such case; the accused was found guilty of causing the death of a woman while attempting to procure the latter's miscarriage. But following the legalisation of abortion in England in 1967, the Irish abortion problem was exported to that jurisdiction and it is estimated that there are in the region of at least 5,000 abortions carried out on Irish women each year in Britain.

There is no legislation governing the performance of a lawful abortion in Ireland, if there truly be such a thing, and there is a movement for a further referendum in 1997 to clarify the position yet again. The difficulties in reconciling the medical and legal definitions of what constitutes abortion make this issue another one on which medical law and ethics may diverge still further (Hogan, 1997). The guidelines from the Medical Council state that 'while the necessity for abortion to preserve the life or health of the sick mother remains to be proved, it is unethical always to withhold treatment beneficial to a pregnant woman, by reason of her pregnancy.'

The right to life is a broad issue for medical law and ethics involving the implementation of protection for the vulnerable in society. The abortion issue remains in a legal limbo following the 1983 constitutional amendment and the X Case. Nobody can be satisfied with such uncertainty.

SUICIDE

Suicide has reached almost epidemic proportions in Ireland with approximately four hundred deaths per year. It is the second most common cause of death in young men aged 15-24. Suicide was much less common in previous decades having an official incidence of 81 deaths in 1971. It has become one of the major public health issues of the 1990s with an official incidence of 383 in 1995. The factors causing this change are many and are deeply rooted in changes in society itself.

Suicide is no longer a crime, but it was only decriminalised in 1993. The National Task Force on Suicide has issued an interim report on suicide and on a prevention strategy (1996). The problem has been recognised as one involving all sectors of the healthcare community, gárdaí, coroners and not least the devastated families of the deceased. The inaugural meeting of the Irish Association of Suicidology in 1996 illustrated the seriousness with which this issue is being taken and the various groups which must play a role in the proposed prevention strategy. The many legal and ethical issues were explored and debated at this open forum (Connolly, 1996). The death of so many people in their productive years is a major challenge to our healthcare system and to society in general.

IN-VITRO FERTILISATION

The matter of assisted reproduction has also emerged as a medico-legal and ethical issue since the 1980s (Warnock Commission, 1984). The Medical Council approves the guidelines promulgated by the Institute of Obstetricians and Gynaecologists of the Royal College of Physicians of Ireland and therapeutic application of in-vitro fertilisation within this framework to married couples is acceptable[16]. However, two major areas of potential difficulty are now apparent. All fertilised embryos produced by the procedure of in-vitro fertilisation should be replaced in the mother's uterus and optimally this should be three in any treatment cycle. The number of embryos produced by ovarian hormonal stimulation varies from one to twelve in typical cases with an average of four. Therefore the question of replacing the surplus embryos arises. The ban on freezing of embryos, present in the 1985 Medical Council Guidelines, has been removed but the many questions arising from embryo storage remain unresolved and have given rise to renewed debate about the legal and ethical problems thus raised (Madden, 1995). Legal restrictions on in-vitro fertilisation show a great diversity throughout Europe (Goldbeck-Wood, 1996) and the problem with poorly drafted legislation leading to the destruction of stored embryos was seen in Britain in the latter part of 1996 (Wise, 1996).

CONTRACEPTION

The area of reproductive medicine has also caused problems for doctors in the area of contraception. The family planning legislation introduced by government in 1979 provided for family planning and for conscientious objection by doctors[17]. However, the greatest difficulty for many doctors and others relates to the prescribing of contraceptives without parental consent to women under seventeen years of age, which is the legal age of consent to sexual intercourse in the Irish jurisdiction. The difficulties were clearly illustrated in the English case of Gillick in which it was held that the rights of the parent are secondary to the rights of the child when that child 'reaches a sufficient understanding and intelligence which would render him capable of making up his own mind'[18]. It is not certain whether an Irish court would adopt the same principle, having regard to the status of the family in the Constitution (Donnelly, 1995).

AMNIOCENTESIS

The availability of amniocentesis is an area of intense discussion and will become a greater issue in the future when combined with increasing sophistication of genetic mapping. The right of parents to know about potential serious illness in their children must be set in the context of both the diagnostic and therapeutic uses of the technique and the ultimate purpose to which it will be put. The dangers to the foetus must also be given full medical, legal and ethical consideration. The care and well-being of children with known or potential physical or mental handicap is an emotive one. Pre-natal diagnosis poses challenges which society must be prepared to meet.

RESEARCH AND CLINICAL TRIALS

Legal and ethical issues arise for consideration in the area of medical research on humans. Such research has always been necessary for the progress of medical science. Evaluation of the efficacy of proposed trials and the risks to the human volunteers participating in them are subject to scrutiny under legislation enacted following the death of a volunteer during a clinical trial in the mid-1980s[19]. Consent for participation in a clinical trial is the only example of true informed consent in this jurisdiction and the criteria are set down in statute[20]. There is also a legal requirement for an ethics committee to give approval for the trial having regard to strict criteria of assessment (Section 8). Ethical codes also set out safeguards for the participants.

ALLOCATION OF SCARCE RESOURCES

All healthcare professionals and managers are experiencing difficulties in deciding where and when to allocate limited resources for patient care. This involves co-operation between the management and clinical teams and cannot be abrogated by either of these teams to be the sole responsibility of the other. Patients have statutory rights under the various Health Acts and yet financial constraints limit the amount of funds available for healthcare. There is both a legal and an ethical obligation on healthcarers to allocate the available resources in accordance with patient needs, efficient use of the funds and in a non-discriminatory manner. This will include active and ongoing review of patient waiting lists by clinicians and managers together and will be a continuing area for medico-legal and ethical problems in future healthcare. Indeed, this may turn out to be one of the most contentious dilemmas to face healthcare in the twenty-first century as patients' expectations and medical technology combine to frustrate financial planners. In Britain, the National Health Service and Community Care Act 1990 established an 'internal market' for health and laid the health services open to litigation concerning allocation of NHS resources (Nedwick, 1993); it has already been the subject of high profile litigation in that jurisdiction. Legal and ethical arguments will centre on what should be considered required and appropriate treatment for a patient, on clinical freedom for doctors and on proper managerial constraints on unnecessary and unsustainable expenditures.

SAFETY AT WORK

A discussion of medical law and ethics as applied to healthcare would not be complete without a brief reference to health and safety at work legislation. This is a proper acknowledgement of the rights of healthcare workers and their patients to work and be treated in a safe and healthy workplace. The legislation enacted since 1989 is one of the most significant advances in public health in the past fifty years. The Barrington Commission Report of 1983 stated that only some 20% of the workforce was covered by the then safety legislation. The healthcare sector was not included in that 20%. There is now a large body of law requiring management to make and keep the workplace safe and to act in a pro-active and preventative way to achieve this. There are statutory duties on employers, employees and others to co-operate in achieving the objectives of workplace safety. Legislation particularly relevant to healthcare workers includes the regulations on manual handling, ionising radiation, carcinogens, biological agents and pregnant employees (HSA, 1993). The enforceable statutory duties of employers to train and give information to healthcare employees will pay dividends in the future wellbeing of workers.

THE FUTURE

All of these many and diverse issues and others are an intrinsic part of the modern healthcare system and lie in the realm of medical law and medical ethics, although they also overlap with other specialities and interests.

The discussion of and teaching of medico-legal and medico-ethical issues must continue to be integrated with clinical teaching and practice for doctors, nurses, other healthcare workers and managers in undergraduate, postgraduate and continuing professional development programmes. There is a continuing requirement for medical law in the broader sense as part of legal education. The ultimate aim is the improvement in delivery of healthcare services to the public.

The government health strategy is underpinned by the key principles of equity, quality of service and accountability (*Shaping a Healthier Future*, 1994). Familiarity with and the application of medical law and medical ethics by healthcare workers will assist in a very positive way in the implementation of these principles in the future.

The increasing number of ethical and legal dilemmas reflects the increasing complexity of medical technology, the emergence of consumer-driven individualism and a serious deficiency of will to address many of the medico-ethical issues out of a misplaced fear of the law and of inability to reach consensus.

Codes of medical law and ethics are not new. Hammurabi of Babylon is credited as being the author of the oldest written code on legislation of medico-legal matters in about 2,000 BC. The Oath of Hippocrates, which is the basis for most codes of medical ethics, dates from about the 4th century BC. But the advances in medical science and technology have opened up a bewildering array of legal and ethical problems with which we are coping poorly at present, although Ireland is not alone in grappling with such problems. Healthcare practitioners have a burdensome duty to consider these issues carefully and insofar as is possible to formulate guidelines on them. These matters cannot be left to the courts alone to decide without the assistance of all qualified bodies and persons. Judges are only specialists and like any other specialists must have the body of knowledge before them to reach properly informed decisions on these medico-legal and ethical questions.

It must also be recognised that there will on occasion be a clear divergence between medical law and medical ethics. This divergence must be kept to the minimum because the common central concern of healthcare and justice is the patient. The principles of doing no harm, of acting for the benefit of the patient and of recognising the value and sanctity of life are ancient ones and as relevant in the 1990s as ever.

The actions of healthcarers must be legal and ethical and yet the individual practitioner must be guided by an informed conscience in each individual case. The richness of the trusting and individual carer-patient relationship must not be lost in any legal and ethical quagmire.

It is now time for the establishment of a Commission on Biomedical Ethics (consisting of all properly interested professional, religious, patient and other groups) to review the medico-ethical issues central to healthcare, only some of which have been addressed briefly in this essay.

REFERENCES

1. Medical Practitioners Act, 1978, section 69(2); Nurses Act, 1985, section 51(2).
2. Bolam v Friern Barnet Management Committee [1957], 2 *All England Reports,* page 118.
3. Sidaway v Governors of Bethlem Royal Hospital [1985] 1 *All England Reports,* page 131.
4. Walsh v Family Planning Services Ltd [1992] 1 *Irish Reports,* page 496.
5. Farrell v Varian. *Medico-Legal Journal of Ireland,* 1990; 1 (1), page 29.
6. Child Care Policy Unit, Department of Health statistics.
7. Child Abuse Guidelines, Department of Health, July 1987; Notification of suspected cases of child abuse between Health Boards and Gardaí, Department of Health, April 1995.
8. Report of the Tribunal of Inquiry into the Blood Transfusion Service Board, Government Publications 1997.
9. Resolution adopted by the 27th World Medical Assembly, Munich, Germany 1973: Medical Data Banks and Computers in Medicine. In – *The Medical Council: A Guide to Ethical Conduct and Behaviour and to Fitness to Practice.* (January 1994) Appendix E.
10. *The Medical Council: A Guide to Ethical Conduct and Behaviour and to Fitness to Practice.* (January 1994). Paragraph 13.01.
11. Report of the Advisory Group on the Transmission of Infectious Diseases in the Health Care Setting. Department of Health, 1997.
12. Re a Word of Court. *Medico-Legal Journal of Ireland,* 1995; 1(2), pages 42-65.
13. BMA guidelines on treatment decisions for patients in persistent vegetative state. Revised July 1996.
14. Vacco v Quill; Compassion in Dying v Washington.
15. Attorney General v X [1992], 1 *Irish Reports,* page 5.
16. *The Medical Council: A Guide to Ethical Conduct and Behaviour and to Fitness to Practice.* (January 1994). Paragraph 40.01 and Appendix G.
17. Health (Family Planning) Act 1979, section 11.
18. Gillick v West Norfolk & Wisbech Area Health Authority [1985] 3 *All England Reports,* page 402.
19. *The Medical Council: A Guide to Ethical Conduct and to Fitness to Practice.* (January 1994), paragraph 41 and appendix H; Royal College of Physicians of Ireland report: *The Use of Drugs in Biomedical Research.* 1986.
20. Control of Clinical Trials Act 1987, section 9.

CHAPTER 13

Nursing and the Health Services

Geraldine McCarthy

INTRODUCTION

This paper will trace the evolution of nursing education and practice from 1947, with the establishment of a separate Department of Health, to 1997. It will highlight present issues and forecast developments which may occur as a result of the *Health Strategy – Shaping a Healthier Future* and the Report on the *Future of Nurse Education and Training*.

GROWTH OF HEALTH SERVICE

This period saw major growth in health and social services with resultant change in nursing. As medicine advanced, the demand for hospital care grew beyond the scope of private charity and increasingly became the concern of the state. Hensey (1993) says: 'The years immediately after the war brought a flood of plans and schemes for development and change of the health services'. Nurses were intimately involved in these developments and changes. Up to 1970 the local authorities operated hospitals side by side with the voluntary hospitals and nursing developed within these institutions.

The 1960s saw a need for health reform. Infectious diseases became less of a problem, but heart disease, cancer and diseases associated with ageing and accidents presented and persist as major concerns. Medicine advanced, and more doctors and nurses began employment in institutional health care settings. The Health Act 1970 established regional health boards and general and specialist regional hospitals developed. These were affiliated to universities, developed as major teaching hospitals for nurses and competed with the voluntary hospitals which were mainly located in Dublin. These hospitals have evolved into very complex work organisations with resultant changes in the role of the nurse.

NUMBER OF NURSES

Today, 27,359 nurses work in the health services. Approximately 12,340 work within hospitals, 1,410 as public health nurses and 8,118 in special facilities (1,005 in midwifery, 923 with sick children, 2,514 with mental handicap clients and 4,576 in psychiatry). If the health services are to be refocused in the community this employment pattern is of concern. The number of registered nurses grew in Ireland to 48,945 registered on the 'live register' in 1994 with a reported 33,344 in active practice of some type (An Bord Altranais, 1995).

Over the years nursing as a career in Ireland has, contrary to the experience of other countries, continued to attract large numbers of highly motivated applicants, far in excess of the number of training places available (McCarthy, 1988). However, with broadening female occupational roles, changes in social structures and in nurse education, nursing may in the future have to compete for students with other occupations. Emigration of Irish nurses continues as a pattern with approximately 1,000 nurses per year seeking validation of qualifications from An Bord Altranais. In general this has been seen as the result of lack of educational opportunities in Ireland, poor prospects of promotion and perceived inadequate remuneration. In future health services, having invested substantially in nurse education, may not be able to afford to continue to allow this skilled resource to be exported.

LEGISLATION

Nursing is regulated by nursing legislation. In 1950 a Nurses Act was introduced to replace the 1919 Act, with the objective of making 'further and better provision for the registration, certification, control and training of nurses and for other matters relating to nurses and the practice of nursing'. This Act established An Bord Altranais which has regulated nurse education and practice since then. The Nurses Act 1985 subsequently gave nurses authority to regulate nursing through a majority of Board members. Powers of the Board have also been extended in areas of training, examination, registration and professional discipline (Nurses Act 1950, 1961, 1985). 1987 saw the establishment of a 'live' register which provides current information on numbers of nurses in the country and individual records. Approximately 2,000 nurses register annually. Presently the Board manages the records of all registered nurses and oversees the education of approximately 4,000 student nurses at any one time. It advises on practice concerns and deals with 'fitness to practice' issues. The Nurses Act 1985 is presently being reviewed. Professional expectations are that the new act will include mandatory post-registration education for all registered nurses and possibly the deletion of the section allowing registration of an ancillary grade.

NURSE EDUCATION AND HOSPITAL INSTITUTIONS

The development of hospital institutions is of vital importance to nursing in general and nurse education in particular. The training of nurses began within hospitals, and training continues to date to be hospital-controlled. In 1947 most nurses were female and unmarried, work hours were long and pay poor. Girls preparing for marriage were recruited to mainly religious training schools and were educated in an apprenticeship manner to supply service for a few years before marriage (Maggs, 1983). This led to the emergence of a hierarchical structure with few experienced nurses and many young apprentices. An exception to this was the psychiatric nursing service, where men were traditionally recruited and employed until retirement. In the 1940s-1950s there were no independent schools of nursing and no developed body of nursing knowledge. There were few nursing tutors and the matron or her assistant taught the trainees at the patient's bedside. The matron knew the character and ability of each probationer. She directed, disciplined, and had no hesitation in advising nurse candidates to leave nursing.

When Florence Nightingale died in 1910 nursing was an emerging profession administered by women and offering nursing and educational opportunities (Deloughery, 1977). Many Irish matrons were educated at St. Thomas's Hospital Nurse Training School, London, established by Nightingale, which became in practice a training school for matrons rather than for nurses. Their education was, according to Abel Smith, permeated by 'the religious zeal of Kaiserwerth, the military discipline of Scutari and the cultural pattern of Ms. Nightingale's Victorian home' (Smith, 1980). Supervision in nurse training extended into all facets of the nurse's life. Living in 'nurses' homes' was essential for practical and economic reasons and for moral and character formation. Trainees were expected to be sober, honest, truthful, punctual, quiet and orderly, clearly and neat, patient, cheerful and kindly (Nightingale, 1952).

It is true to say that Ms. Nightingale's ideas of vocation, discipline, diligence and obedience lived on in Irish nursing up to the 1970s and some remnants may still remain. They were perpetrated through an outdated method of education which included personal training and schools of nursing set within the hospital culture. The effects can be seen within the profession itself and in social appreciation and expectation. They have affected professional growth, and inhibited roles, education, accountability and management.

DEVELOPING HEALTH SERVICES

As the health services developed, the need to recruit and train nurses to staff the growing number of hospitals became paramount. This saw the development of separate nurse training programmes in the public and voluntary sector, and in disciplines such as psychiatry, paediatrics and mental handicap. It is difficult to identify which hospitals had training schools with formal hours of tuition in 1947. In 1950 twenty-five general hospitals offered training in an apprentice mode and by 1980 the number of schools had grown to seventy-two (Dept. of Health, 1980). In 1980 the Working Party on General Nursing recommended rationalisation to a total of fifteen schools. This rationalisation has occurred and today the number has been reduced to forty-four (eighteen in general, nine in psychiatry, three in sick children, seven each in mental handicap and midwifery) (An Bord Altranais, 1995). It is thought possible that, as schools affiliate with universities, a further reduction in the number of schools will occur.

TRAINING REQUIREMENTS

A directive from An Bord Altranais in 1957 stated that a preliminary training school would be an essential requirement in any hospital which trained student nurses by 1960. In June 1966 the Board further stipulated that all students should have a minimum of eighteen to twenty-two weeks' formal instruction; the block system of protected study time was introduced (An Bord Altranais, 1957, 1966) and formal schools were set up within hospitals. Facilities varied from purpose-build schools to converted accommodation. The matron of the hospital was in charge of the school and the post of principal tutor, created in 1969, carried varying degrees of authority and autonomy.

Over the years considerable changes have occurred in the number of hours spent in attending formal lectures, the type of material presented and the range of clinical experience gained. Since Ireland became a member of the European Union, Irish nurses are affected by decisions taken by that body. The two general nursing directives 77/452/EEC and 77/453/EEC were agreed by the Council of Ministers and signed on 27 June 1979. These had to be implemented by June 1979 and so a commitment was made to introduce change to the education of nurses. Subsequently midwifery directives were applied by directive 80/155/EEC. The directives are concerned with mutual recognition of formal qualification of nurses responsible for care, and aim to ensure a comparatively high standard of training of nursing personnel throughout the Community. To comply with the general directives, student nurse training was extended into areas of obstetrics, paediatrics, geriatrics, psychiatry and community care. There are currently no European Community directives for mental handicap, psychiatry or sick children's nurse training programmes.

Supplementary registers have meant that nurses qualifying in one branch of nursing and wishing to pursue study in another area must, up to the present time, undertake two or more extra years' training even though there is a common core of knowledge in all branches. It has appeared over the years that hospitals not only have a vested interest in a long training, but that they also have a financial stake in the fragmentation of training. To gain wide experience means being a poorly paid temporary employee for years.

The form of nurse education legalised in the 1919 Nurses Act was further authenticated by the legislation of 1950. It was a compromise based on the existing hospital system and continued to exist in Ireland until 1994 when reforms were introduced. It produced nurses who were highly skilled at hospital work but were unquestioning and submissive (Treacy, 1987). Davies says: 'the strategy of nurse education meant the staffing of hospitals with a strictly disciplined labour force of probationers; they would do the work of the hospital both uncomplaining and cheaply' (Davies, 1980). The system neither challenged the other health care professions nor made demands on administration. It could only have existed in a world where women were prepared to be self-denying, hard-working and amenable to discipline.

UNIVERSITY EDUCATION

Despite criticisms since the 1940s, the system of nurse education in operation in Ireland continued until 1994 (McGowan, 1979; O'Dwyer, 1984). In June 1973 a degree course of four years for student nurses was proposed in University College Galway (UCG, unpublished). Bord Altranais supported the establishment of the degree course (An Bord Altranais, 1973) but regrettably this development did not occur. The 1980 Working Party on General Nursing recommended a 'common basic training' where students of all disciplines of nursing would study similar material together. In 1984 Bord Altranais took a policy decision that nursing education should move into universities and institutes of higher education. In 1994, after four years of deliberation and consultations (An Bord Altranais, 1991), a review body which represented nurses, An Bord Altranais, health boards, the Higher Educational Authority and the National Council for Educational Awards reported its findings on nurse education to the Department of Health (An Bord Altranais, 1994). The recommendations were for change at basic and post-basic levels, with the introduction of diplomas and degrees and academic accreditation for all courses. These recommendations were endorsed in the *Health Strategy:* 'it is necessary to align the regime for nurse education more closely with the demands of a modern day health service'. Nurses welcomed the contents and appreciated the need to produce a body of nurse researchers and reflective thinkers who will help all nurses to ask questions about nursing.

In October 1994, Galway University Hospital School of Nursing in collaboration with University College Galway introduced the first diploma programme for student nurses studying general nursing. In 1995 and 1996 eleven other hospital schools in collaboration with an associated third level college offered the diploma (Byrne, 1997). It is intended that all other schools will be included by 1998. Two specialist schools in psychiatry have also entered the new format of education through a common foundation programme. The future of mental handicap nurse training is still under review, and nurse training for sick children has become a post-registration qualification.

The change has meant supernumerary status for student nurses, with student involvement in clinical areas to gain experience rather than to give service; a grant rather than a salary, extension of the theoretical component and teaching of specialist subjects in the biological and social sciences by university departments, access to a one-year degree programme and replacement of students in the workforce by qualified nurses and other workers. However, students will still remain in schools of nursing for most of their education, have little opportunity to mix with other college students and will work at least a thirty-hour week, making them significantly different from all other third level students.

Up to recently, each hospital school of nursing (while using An Bord Altranais criteria as guidelines) set its own standards of entry, advertised, interviewed and recruited students. This created many difficulties for potential students, parents, teachers and administrators and resulted in a system which was inefficient and expensive. In 1973 An Bord Altranais introduced minimum educational standards which are updated regularly. In 1994, when the first diploma programme was introduced, a centralised system of application and selection for nurse training was established. It is possible that this Nursing Application Centre will amalgamate with the Central Applications Office for other third level places in the future.

ISSUES TO BE ADDRESSED

The reforms of nurse education have been influenced by international trends and by the fact that the nurse was the only member of the health care team not receiving a university education. The Department of Health is to be complimented in the speed of introduction of reform but a number of issues remain to be addressed. There is the challenge of establishing departments of nursing within third level institutions, staffed and headed by nurses. At present it appears that there are not enough Irish nurses with appropriate and acceptable university teaching and research experience to head up these departments. This is due to the lack of proactive planning by the professions, and the lack of scholarships or state aid to nurses who could have gained this experience in departments of nursing in countries where nurse education had already been developed.

The number of nurse teachers in the country has always been small and although numbers have increased over the years to 295 on the 1995 register, the wastage to nurse administration has been considerable. It appears that from an economic and role point of view, teaching was not an attractive progression in nursing for many well-qualified and motivated nurses (McGowan, 1979; Dept. of Health, 1980). Since 1966 most nurse tutors have held National University of Ireland Diplomas in Nurse Teaching and since 1988 all tutors registering with An Bord Altranais hold a Bachelor of Nursing. Having completed the primary degree, many nurse teachers have taken masters' degrees, mostly in education. There is a possibility that two types of teachers of nursing will now evolve, those based in the schools of nursing and those in academic departments, with different terms of employment and responsibility. Careful consideration needs to be given to developing joint appointments between the nursing and education services, and between hospital schools and university nursing departments. The question of funded chairs of nursing also needs to be addressed so that nursing has the same status and entitlements in universities as all other disciplines.

Other issues relate to student nurses as university students rather than Department of Health students such as curriculum; student grants; location of schools of nursing; common core generalist training versus specialist training from the beginning. Finally, the challenge of the amalgamation of the entire nurse education system into the university as offered in other countries will have to be addressed.

SUPPORT WORKERS AND SKILL MIX

In the 1970s pressure was exerted on An Bord Altranais to introduce a second grade of nurse, primarily to offset shortage of nursing personnel. An Bord Altranais did not accede to this request (An Bord Altranais, 1970, 1973), but recommended to the Minister that an in-depth study of nurse training be undertaken. This was carried out in 1975-1980, but The Working Party Report on General Nursing did not recommend a second grade of nurse. In the changes taking place in nurse education today, other grades of workers are being introduced into the workforce to work side by side with nurses. It is anticipated that these will grow in number and will lead to problems relating to skill mix which have not previously been encountered in Irish nursing. Employing authorities should note that skill mix initiatives have failed elsewhere from a quality of care perspective, and a return of almost full professional nurse staffing has been achieved in many of the major hospitals and health care agencies throughout the world.

POST-REGISTRATION EDUCATION AND SPECIALISATION

Over the years Irish nurses have continued to study after receiving a first qualification, and one of the most frequent requests from registered nurses is for continuing education. Traditionally this has meant studying for a second registration with An Bord Altranais. The most popular choice has been midwifery, as nurses anticipate its need for public health nursing and even for positions as matrons of district hospitals. Other than this there was very little post-basic nurse education provided by either employing authorities or An Bord Altranais in the 1950s and 1960s. Nurses aspiring to university education or specialist study have had to travel to the universities of England or Scotland. This must be explained partly by a lack of understanding or commitment to in-service or ongoing education, and partly by a lack of nurse leaders, primarily educationalist, to plan and co-ordinate such courses. Professional organisations have united to campaign for university education.

A major step in the promotion of post-basic nursing education was the establishment of the Nurse Tutor Diploma Course in University College Dublin in 1960 and the Diploma in Public Health Nursing in 1986. These remained the only graduate diplomas in nursing until 1988, when a degree for nurse teachers was introduced. In 1974 a Faculty of Nursing in The Royal College of Surgeons of Ireland was established (Crowley, 1982). It has over the years fulfilled a need evidenced by the large attendance at courses offered in specialist subject areas. From the 1970s onwards hospitals and other employing authorities seconded individuals to the growing number of available courses and in this way provided expert nurses to teach others.

In 1990 University College Dublin led the way in establishing a part-time degree level programme for registered nurses. University College Cork followed in 1994 and Dublin City University in 1996, and today the number of graduates is growing. The Higher Diploma in Public Health Nursing is available at University College Cork and University College Dublin. Midwifery programmes are being awarded diploma status in a number of universities and Trinity College offers a Diploma/Masters Degree in Care of the Elderly. Another interesting development has been the increasing number of Irish nurses who are taking time away from the practice of their profession to pursue full-time third-level degree courses in education, psychology, sociology, law, social policy, child care, public administration etc. Since the introduction of the reforms in student nurse training, increasing numbers of registered nurses have begun to study for degrees. This has led to considerable difficulty for those who must combine family and work commitments with a student role. It appears that only some nurses will have the time or energy or desire to upgrade their qualifications. This may lead to difficulties in the workplace, with some graduates and some non-graduates all performing the same work.

As nurses strive to gain graduate status, challenges will face both service providers and educationalists. If service providers require expert nurses to address the areas identified in the health strategy such as cancer care, cardio-vascular disease, accidents, the elderly, public health and health promotion, will they help nurses attain the appropriate update to their education to function in these areas, or will they expect nurses to do so totally on their own? For university nursing heads of departments, the challenge will be to provide these courses in a user-friendly, cost-effective, full- or part-time and focused manner to meet the needs of the health services. Other specialist courses are provided directly in hospitals and the challenge for the future will be to integrate these into third level education.

NURSING PRACTICE

Over the years under review the role of the nurse has changed substantially. The contribution of the religious orders to nursing practice cannot be underestimated (Bolster, 1982; Butler, 1984). They have played a significant part in emphasising the plight of the sick, the poor and the need for human dignity in health care. They have also helped in elevating the status of women and of nurses. However, the vocational, self-sacrificing, hierarchical emphasis which permeated the profession has not been to the advantage of a predominantly female workforce who until recently were poorly organised and recognised. A major change now taking place in religious orders is the lack of vocations, with a resultant loss of religious sisters and brothers in hospitals. What is interesting is that the religious orders which grew out of community need produced many nurses who firmly established themselves until recently in nursing management roles. However, we are now seeing a return to the community, with many orders again taking up the plight of the homeless, the alcoholic, the drug dependent and the traveller, and leading the way for nursing and for the health service.

SEXUAL DIVISION OF LABOUR

The sexual division of labour is important in nursing (Davies, 1972; Scanlon, 1991). In the nineteenth century, women were excluded from the labour market by factory acts, legal prohibitions and trade practices. Married nurses were discouraged from working until the lifting of the marriage bar in the 1970s. This ideology perceived women and men as naturally different, with abilities suited to different spheres of employment. Nursing today still figures predominantly as a female occupation. The profession suffered a shortage of nurses in the seventies (Hanrahan, 1975) in 1975 and felt the 'experience drain', and many nurse managers say the same is happening today. However, since the lifting of the marriage bar, married nurses in increasing numbers continue to work and are available for more part-time employment, which is reflected in the composition of the labour force. Today, as the number of nurses in training is reduced, a shortage of registered nurses may again be experienced, or nursing may experience significant difficulties in retaining those trained in the workforce. It may be that registered nurses will have to be empowered to work through still more flexible hiring arrangements and more 'back to nursing' educational programmes.

CHANGING ROLE OF THE NURSE

Growth in knowledge since 1947 has changed the role of the nurse. Advances in medical science, diagnosis and investigation, treatment modalities, organ and tissue transplantation have contributed to this change, and to the development of the specialist nurse. Nursing today is performing many of the procedures formerly carried out by medical colleagues, in support of the advancement of scientific knowledge and technology. Factors which are also changing the role are: more rapid patient turnover and emphasis on cost, complexity of procedures undertaken, enlightened, demanding and litigation-conscious patients, social and economic problems, the 1991 Child Care Act, anticipatory care of the elderly especially in rural situations, and deinstitutionalisation of patients previously housed in psychiatric settings. The challenges of substance abuse, increasing numbers of the aged, health problems associated with unemployment, cardio-vascular disease, cancers and accidents, together with an emphasis on quality, social gain and accountability, demand a change in emphasis for nursing to a more community-based health service.

As described previously, most general nurses still work in acute or long-stay hospitals. Within these many have developed specialist roles, for example renal nurse, diabetic nurse specialist, stomatherapist, incontinence advisor, critical care nurse, palliative care nurse, oncology nurse, behaviour therapist etc. The requirements for these highly-trained nurses will always persist and even today there is a failure in many hospitals to fill positions in speciality areas such as theatres and intensive care units, despite multiple advertisements. Indeed it may be that specialist nursing roles need to be extended further and that many more nurse-led clinics should be available, with independent practitioners holding prescribing rights. However, many nurses also work in hospitals in a generalist mode. In the future these will need to be more skilled to expedite diagnostic or treatment protocols and to partake in proactive discharge planning with community services where necessary.

Up until the mid-twentieth century, mental health provision was primarily institution-based and custodial in nature (Dept. of Health, 1966). The role of the psychiatric nurses was to maintain order and to protect the patient and the public (Henry, 1989). A number of important changes including updated Mental Treatment Legislation (Dept. of Health, 1995) and pharmacological advances led to plans for the service whereby patients were treated in general hospitals, in day care centres or at home (Dept. of Health, 1984). Thus psychiatric nurses were enabled to develop new roles and many of the 4,576 psychiatric nurses work today in community services. Mental handicap nursing has developed; 2,514 mental handicap nurses work in educative-supportive and sometimes long-term care giver roles.

Many nurses work with the elderly in institutional settings and care of the elderly has changed considerably (Dept. of Health, 1988). The number of nurses caring for the aged may need to be increased, especially in light of the Nursing Home Act, and nurses caring for the elderly in the future may need to develop new skills to cope with the increasingly elderly population and their demand for a range of services. In many long-stay hospitals a more specialised form of nursing has been developed with the aim of maintaining maximum levels of independence, physical and cognitive functioning. This may need further development over time. Consideration should also be given to establishing low-cost nurse-administered units with respite beds, and day services and nurses should have the assessment, admission and discharge rights to ensure a smooth movement of patients to and from the community nursing services. Midwifery has continued to evolve as a separate entity and most midwives work in hospital services. A few domiciliary midwives practice independently. As demand increases, domiciliary midwifery services may need expansion.

PUBLIC HEALTH NURSING

The earliest community nursing was delivered by midwives and the present system of public health nursing which employs 1,410 nurses had its origins in the dispensary system, the Health Act 1953, and a White Paper of 1966 which outlined the direction for future developments in public health nursing. The role of the public health nurse in the 1990s results from an amalgamation of three distinct specialist areas of community nursing: domiciliary midwifery, public health nursing, and nursing care of sick people at home. The role of the public health nurse today incorporates elements of these three areas. Under section 102 of the 1947 Health Act, provision was made for a nursing service to any person requiring advice and assistance on matters relating to health and assistance at home. At this time a home nursing service was provided by religious orders, and voluntary organisations including the Queen Victoria Jubilee Institute for Nurses and the Lady Dudley Nursing Scheme. The midwifery service continued to operate separately until the Health Act 1953 when these services were amalgamated with local authorities. Subsequently many of the dispensary midwives who had general nursing qualifications undertook a short course in public health nursing and were then appointed as full-time public health nurses. Through the amalgamation of public health nursing, midwifery and home nursing services, the potential was created for one nurse working in the community to provide a comprehensive public health nursing service, which is the manner in which the service is organised today.

Although in 1956 the Minister of Health encouraged health authorities to make available home nursing and midwifery services, a ministerial circular was not issued until 1966 (Dept. of Health, 1966). This circular outlined the aims and objectives of the service and indicated the various client groups with whom the public health nurse should work. It also recommended the appointment of superintendent public health nurses wherever ten or more nurses were employed. The senior public health nursing position was established in 1982. Until 1987 An Bord Altranais provided training for public health nurses. Today a one-year full-time academic programme leading to a higher diploma in public health nursing and registration as a public health nurse is available at both University College Cork and University College Dublin.

Many reports, but in particular *The Commission of Health Funding, Health the Wider Dimension, Planning for the Future, Working Party on Workload of Public Health Nurses, Survey of the Workload of Public Health Nurses* and *Shaping a Healthier Future* have implications for extending the public health nursing service. However, the system has considerable difficulties in relation to case-load, generalist functions and lack of support services, especially in rural areas. Numerous special reports and evaluations of the public health nursing service have been undertaken since 1976, including one by Burke (1986) which identified dimensions of the public health nurse's role. The most recent report by Sullivan identifies role, links with other services and professions and the issue of professional specialism as the most pertinent concerns (Sullivan, 1995).

There is no doubt that the public health nursing service is a comprehensive and satisfactory one despite case load diversity and limited resources. However, the public health element of the role is not used to its best capacity due to pressure of other work. If community services are to be developed, more nurses must work in the community. Some of these must be public health nurses who have the education and position within society to deliver on many of the targets outlined in the *Health Strategy* four-year action plan relating to health promotion, women's health, family planning, child health etc. More general nurses with diverse experiences and pertinent education should also be employed to work with the aged and the acute or chronic sick in their homes. Whether there is a potential to deploy general nurses as suggested in the *Report of the Commission on Health Funding* requires further investigation.

POSTS OF RESPONSIBILITY

Finally, in relation to roles perhaps one of the most dramatic developments has been the change in the role of the matron/chief nurse. Traditionally the supervisor of many departments and functions and teacher of nurses, the matron's function has today evolved into a very complex one which few understand and for which nurses have not been prepared. It appears that the work will become even more complicated, requiring new skills and knowledge.

Within the health service changes to date, a professional problem for nurses is that they have not been able to articulate their work or claim responsibility for many of the excellent health care outcomes which they have brought about. Many nurses who want to be treated as professional workers are unprepared educationally, and often unwilling, to take on the full responsibilities which go with independence and autonomy in practice. Those who work in hospitals have been indoctrinated into collective responsibility; some are now finding it difficult to take on primary nursing with its individual client relationship and accountability, and prefer to work in the traditional task-orientated manner. For those nurses who are educated and willing to take on a more extensive and responsible role, there is frequent opposition from other health care professionals who want the nurse to remain subservient.

ORGANISED NURSES

Many organisations have been established over the years to aid nurses to achieve their objectives. Amongst these are the Irish Matrons Association and more recently a number of trade unions: Irish Nurses' Organisation, SIPTU, IMPACT and Psychiatric Nurses' Association. The Irish Nurses' Organisation grew from The Irish Nurses' Union, which was formed in 1919, and remains the largest organisation representing nurses in Ireland. The organisation has grown throughout the years in membership and activity in professional and educational domains. Its activities reflect the growing concern of nurses for their profession, and the extension of their interests and capabilities. Through the organisation Irish nurses are represented on the International Council of Nurses and in this way are linked to international nursing. The Irish Matrons' Association, formed in 1904, continues to represent the views of nurse administrators.

CONCLUSION

This paper has presented the changes and evolution in the education, training and working practices of nurses in the past fifty years. It shows how societal and health care change and legislation have affected the role of the nurse and progression to a self-governing and self-disciplining profession. The paper also describes the problems which still need to be addressed: the implications for nurses of increasing community care services and shortened hospital stays; the attempts being made to reorganise and broaden nurse education so that nurses can deliver a broader spectrum of care in hospital and in the community, and to clarify and develop the content of nursing and produce nurse researchers. It is contended that in the future a greater number of nurses will be required to work in the community and more highly specialised nurses to work in hospitals, with more focused management to expedite specialist diagnosis and treatment.

The author firmly believes that nursing has a vital role to play in the health services of the future and in implementing the proposals for health care reform. Nurses are seen as major contributors to health, and nursing will continue to be an attractive profession as it plays such a vital role in caring for the sick, the injured and in providing personal satisfaction which goes well beyond the material. On reflecting back over the past half century and taking note of both the past and present accomplishments, the author is acutely aware of the fact that nurses have not played any really major leadership role in health care policy. However, nursing is one of the two great comprehensive health disciplines; it is the partner of medicine on the cure-care team.

Both the public and the discipline of nursing have paid a high price for the fact that nurses, in their zeal to improve the clinical care of the hospitalised sick, allowed both nursing education and practice to become largely hospital-based and until recently medicine-dominated. The fact is that nursing in itself is therapeutic and should be available to people when they need it regardless of where they are or whether a doctor is involved in care, but this has been forgotten in the push to develop medical knowledge and skills, technology, cure and cost-effectiveness. If nursing had advanced side by side with medicine and at the same pace over the past fifty years, many of the problems which now beset the Irish health services might have been avoided. Failure to recognise that nursing is a discrete health discipline may have led to the underdevelopment of self-care as compared to cure. It also may be one of the major reasons why present health services are increasingly unsatisfactory to the public, costly, and mainly concentrated in institutions rather than the community.

Reasons why it has taken so long for the real nature of nursing to be clearly defined, understood and accepted include: the fact that most nurses were and are women; the failure of nurses to use the power available to them; the persistence and success with which nurses, doctors and others have fought to keep nursing education in hospital-dominated schools and outside of universities and institutions of higher learning; and that nurses have allowed themselves to become in the main acquiescent participants and unquestioning health care workers.

Looking into the future, nurses must establish themselves as truly independent, autonomous practitioners accountable directly to their peers and the persons whom they serve. They must be able to provide nursing care in institutions and in the community, wherever the client is, without recourse to another health profession. They must take their place as members of decision-making groups which deal with national, regional and local health and related policies, and became visible participants in all aspects of the health services. Nursing exists to assist individuals and groups to optimise and integrate physical, mental and social functions. Nurses have served the health service well during the last fifty years and will continue to do so.

CHAPTER 14

Management and the Health Professional

Patricia Brown and Geoffrey Chadwick

This paper is informed by an analysis of twenty-nine in-depth interviews with Irish hospital consultants working in Dublin public voluntary hospitals. The research was undertaken by Patricia Brown as part of a PhD programme with Brunel University.

Management, in the context of a state-funded professional services area such as health, is a complex multi-level activity. There are no readily available management blueprints that can be applied off the shelf within all health care systems. On the contrary, the current international health management literature contains as much contention as agreement on appropriate ways of managing health services. There is consensus, however, on the importance of strengthening the management capacity of health care systems.

This paper is a modest contribution to policy thinking in this important area. The focus is necessarily narrow: 'health professional' in the context of the article refers to medical consultants working in the acute hospital sector. We draw upon research based on the views of consultants working in the public voluntary sector to substantiate and support our understanding of the issues. The purpose of our contribution is to explore the issue of management and the medical consultants with specific reference to the Irish health service context. The context refers to the nature of the Irish health system, how it developed, how much direct control the state now has, and what is the current policy for hospitals.

INTRODUCTION

Since the 1980s, health policymakers in most Organisation of Economic Co-operation and Development (OECD) countries have been immersed in the process of health system reform, adjustment and change. The pressures for change are readily identifiable and common across health care systems. The main difficulties countries face are in financing health expenditure and containing its growth. Their concerns emerge in the context of

* the ageing of OECD populations;

* the development and growth of expensive medical technology;

* rising expectations about standards of medical care.

While these factors are outside the control of policy, others that contribute to health expenditure growth are not. In their 1992 Report *The Reform of Health Care*, the OECD identified some important factors that are within the competence of government to address:

* inappropriate financial incentives for providers;

* harmful monopolistic and restrictive practices exercised by providers;

* unsuitable organisational and management structures;

* poorly designed regulatory mechanisms;

* remediable gaps in information about effectiveness and costs (OECD 1992, 17).

These are factors that governments in OECD countries have focused attention on. It is evident from this list that provider behaviour is a significant concern, given the important resource allocation decisions that doctors make within health care systems. While broad agreement exists on some of the key factors that contribute to reducing efficiency and effectiveness, there is less consensus on the strategies and techniques that are likely to improve health system performance. Given the differences in the institutional character of health care systems, this is not surprising. The contribution of the different factors identified above will vary by country.

The purpose of the analysis that follows is to address the factors that contribute in positive or negative ways to the efficient and effective management of clinical practice at hospital level in Ireland. The initial section provides a review of the development of the Irish hospital system and health policy for hospitals from 1950-1970s. The objective here is to identify the crucial historical factors that shaped the cultural and hospital policy in Ireland over that period, the nature of the state's response and its capacity to meet the challenge of effectively developing and co-ordinating the public hospital system. The period from the late 1970s to the 1990s marks a distinct policy phase in Irish health care policy, and the results of the analysis of a survey of Irish hospital consultants working in joint board and public voluntary hospitals in Dublin are discussed, in the context of changes in health policy for hospitals.

The final section of the paper looks to the future. Some of the principles that might guide the formulation of health policy for hospitals are identified, and justified with reference to the preceding analysis.

DEVELOPMENT OF PUBLICLY-FUNDED HOSPITAL SERVICES

The health services in the 1950s were a vast improvement on those which existed in the early 1940s. Tuberculosis and other infectious diseases had been brought under control. Services for mothers and babies were greatly improved and maternal and infant mortality reduced significantly in a short time. Modern hospital and specialist treatment was made available at nominal or no charge to the majority of the population on the principle that the state had a responsibility for those who could not afford to pay for hospital treatment. The VHI protected those not covered by public schemes... In the space of a dozen years, Ireland had developed a modern health service which compared favourably with those of more prosperous countries (Barrington 1987, 248-9).

The 1950s marked the beginning of a significant period in the development of Irish health services, when the role and responsibility of the Irish state for health care expanded. New compromises had been worked out with the various interests involved, facilitating the transition from a system based largely on charitable and private medicine, with a residual state service, to a publicly provided system that guaranteed service as of right to the majority of the population.

When one focuses on the development of the state-funded hospital services over the period 1940-1970, one can still identify a legacy from the earlier period that accounts for some important features of state health policy for hospitals in the period up to the 1970s.

THE POOR LAW LEGACY

The origin of the state hospital system in the poor law is particularly significant in Ireland. Following the 1838 Poor Relief Act, a total of 163 workhouses were established with the primary role of providing shelter for the destitute. The workhouses also included some ward provisions for their sick inmates which were later improved and opened to sick persons outside the destitute class. The workhouses were funded by local taxation (the Poor Rate) which also met the cost of a new district dispensary system and certain public health provisions. Institutions established under the poor law, even as they were upgraded and converted into county hospitals, district hospitals and county homes during the present century, carried a cultural/historical legacy that was difficult to overcome. Generally they were perceived in a very negative light by physicians, patients and the general population. The very low level of funding provided for these institutions during the nineteenth and early twentieth centuries contributed to a negative image of state institutions among both the profession and the general population.

> In some cases the change of name was accompanied by a change
> of attitude but to many old people admission to the 'poorhouse' was
> still a fate too horrible to contemplate (Fleetwood, 1983, 168-9).

The poor law and its institutions in the nineteenth century were as much instruments of social control (containing the spread of disease and segregating the sick from the healthy) as they were a response to the health and social needs of the poorer sections of Irish society (Robins, 1980; Powell, 1989). The poor law was to all intents and purposes a system of last resort.

In the absence of significant developments in medical science and public health knowledge, the public hospital system played little more than a containment/custodial role. The Commission on Health Funding describes the situation thus :

> Hospitals had been places of last resort for the poor whose housing
> or family circumstances were so bad that they did not permit even
> a minimum standard of nursing care. Those who could afford to pay
> for medical and nursing care were treated at home. (Department of
> Health, 1987, 33).

This all changed with developments in medical knowledge that helped to bring contagious diseases under control. Hospitals became much safer environments for the care and treatment of the sick.

STATE INVOLVEMENT: THE IRISH HOSPITAL SWEEPSTAKES

By the 1930s the need and demand for hospital care exceeded the capacity of the existing hospital system. The public voluntary hospitals, which were at that time the main teaching and treatment centres, provided the highest technical standard of care. The state hospitals (mainly former workhouses) were generally of much poorer quality, as the following excerpt from the *Report of the Commission on Health Funding* suggests: '. . . the standard of accommodation and the quality of service owed more to the concepts of the poor law than to modern thinking on medical care' (Department of Health, 1987, 33).

As a consequence of the growing demand for their services the public voluntary hospitals found it increasingly difficult to resource, from their investment income and from donations, the cost of treatment for the poor, and consequently their reliance on private practice grew. The establishment by the public voluntary hospitals of the Sweepstakes was in response to the growing funding crisis. The Sweepstakes was a tremendous success and, coupled with the intervention of the state in establishing the Hospital Commission to adjudicate on the distribution of the fund, was an important development. So also was the decision to allocate money for the development and upgrading of rural local authority hospitals. Although Barrington notes the Commission's lack of success in rationalising the hospital system, it did nonetheless provide for the first time a comprehensive framework for the co-ordination and planning of publicly funded hospital services.

1940–1966

Through the 1940s and 1950s state responsibility for health expenditure increased. This was also a period of intense ideological debate about the direction health policy should take. It was a debate about the respective roles of market-based private practice and publicly-funded health care provision, and the extent and nature of the state's responsibility for the co-ordination and planning of a publicly-funded service.

Eligibility for hospital services was extended to the majority, but not to the entire population. The state accepted that the provision of a national health service free to everybody at the point of use was not at that time realistic. This was reiterated in 1966. This in turn met the professionals' concerns that they would have an alternative to state practice; limiting eligibility for public hospital services protected private practice. The role and independence of public voluntary hospitals were also protected, with the state conceding the choice of hospital and consultant to public patients. The state also compromised on the question of medical education, and allowed public voluntary hospitals to continue as major medical education centres along with the universities. The restrictions on eligibility for the mother and child scheme and the school health scheme protected both the private practice base of the profession and the public voluntary hospitals, and undoubtedly strengthened their respective positions. The founding of the VHI in 1955, and the extension of the right to private practice to local government hospital surgeons, further protected the private health sector.

Reforms introduced under the 1947 and 1953 Health Acts did help to streamline and more clearly designate the responsibility of the new Department of Health and the local authorities (Hensey, 1992, 42). It soon became apparent, however, that the size of the administrative unit (the county) was too small for the effective planning of the acute hospital services, as Hensey explains:

> . . . for the general organisation of hospital services, the county had become too small a unit in 1966; over half of all in-patients in acute hospitals in the larger centres and specialist services at out-patient departments were organised increasingly on a regional basis . . . For many counties, hundreds of patients were being sent annually at the expense of the local authority to hospital in other areas, but in these circumstances, the county concerned had no say in the organisation or operation of the hospital. (Hensey, 1992, 58).

The system of local administration in place up to the 1970s, despite reform, had clearly not kept pace with changes and developments in the public hospital system. The White Paper, *The Health Services and their Further Development*, 1966, signalled the government's intention to regionalise health administration by grouping counties into health board areas under the central direction of the Department of Health. It also announced the removal of the last vestiges of the poor law by the ending of the dispensary system and its replacement by a choice of doctor scheme. These measures were implemented by the Health Act 1970.

THE FITZGERALD REPORT

A working party was established in 1967 to review the general hospital system, under a medical consultant in one of the major Dublin public voluntary hospitals. The Fitzgerald Report, named after the chairman, recognised the essential role of planning and co-ordinating in supporting and facilitating the provision of high quality hospital care. The Report's acknowledgement of the need for mechanisms to co-ordinate both health board and public voluntary hospital services was an important development, given the rivalries between health board and public voluntary hospitals. The willingness of consultants to lay aside institutional differences to reach shared conclusions on key policy issues for the hospital sector as a whole was itself an achievement.

The Fitzgerald Report recommended a significant reduction in the number of acute general hospitals. Larger hospitals were favoured on grounds of safety, medical and nursing training and economics. The report also advocated the establishment of regional structures to oversee hospital services; it supported the integrated planning of health board and public voluntary hospital services; and it accepted the need to co-ordinate general practitioner and hospital care. The Report generated controversy at the time and only a few of its principal findings were implemented, but it remained nonetheless a landmark report in the history of Irish health policy. It signalled an era of partnership between the Department of Health, the medical profession and the voluntary hospitals. Generally the 1970s stands out as as a period when the medical profession were facilitated in making an input into policy formation through their participation in health boards, working groups, and advisory bodies such as Comhairle na nOspidéal, the establishment of which had been recommended by the Fitzgerald Report.

GROWTH IN EXPENDITURE

Health expenditure grew rapidly between 1960 and 1980, from 3.2 % of GNP in 1960 to 8.3% in the early 1980s (Department of Health, 1989, 42). By 1977 exchequer funding accounted for 94.5 % of total health costs (Department of Health 1989, 40). Public expenditure was then under review in Ireland, as in most OECD countries. The severe world recession, combined with over a decade of rising public expenditure (funded in many countries through deficit borrowing), rising unemployment, and ageing populations, was giving cause for concern about the ability of governments to sustain social expenditure levels.

A period of retrenchment followed, and Ireland was no exception. However, the magnitude of the decline in Irish health expenditure in the period 1980-90 was remarkable in an OECD context (OECD 1992). The health cuts in Ireland were achieved mainly by reducing hospital expenditure. In the period 1980-88, expenditure on hospital services declined by nearly 15%. In the same period, according to Wiley and Fetter:

there was a twenty per cent decline in acute hospital beds, a nineteen per cent decline in average length of stay, a twenty-five percent decline in hospital bed days produced and just a five per cent decline in discharges from the acute hospital system (Wiley and Fetter, xii).

By 1988 Irish patterns of use of in-patient care were well within the OECD averages and, in some instances, our indicators were much lower, as for example in the case of beds per 1000 inhabitants and the average length of stay (Schrieber *et al*, 1991, 23-28). However a NESC report in 1993 found Irish ratios of bed occupancy per 1000 population were considerably higher than for United Kingdom countries (England, Wales, Scotland and Northern Ireland), and that the acute bed/population ratio for Ireland was above the average of England and Wales. The study concluded that there was in 1979 an over-provision of acute hospital beds in Ireland (NESC, 1983, 39).

The cuts in health, particularly hospital, expenditure resulted in lengthening waiting lists for public hospital care by the 1980s. Those who could afford private care appear to have taken this option, given the substantial increase in VHI subscriptions during this period (Nolan, 1991).

THE COMMISSION ON HEALTH FUNDING, 1989

Public concern and dissatisfaction with the health services surfaced during the 1987 general election campaign. The across-the-board cuts introduced in the early and mid-1980s proved to be a rather crude strategy and highlighted the need for a rigorous review. The Commission on Health Funding was established in 1987. Its analysis revealed weaknesses in the planning, organisation management and administration of the system which reduced the efficiency, effectiveness and responsiveness of the system, apart altogether from the funding level.

Much of the commission's analysis focused upon the hospital services. And given the background to the commission's report, it is not surprising that questions of equity and access emerged as important issues. The commission noted with concern the public perception of a hospital system where 'access to the public acute hospital system' was viewed as 'seriously inequitable' (Department of Health 1989, 238). The commission accepted that this perception had some basis in fact when it acknowledged that:

The rationing system in place in acute hospitals is based to some extent on ability to pay and, indeed, to some extent on arbitrary criteria, such as accidents of geography or timing, or indeed even personal persistence. It is inequitable that patients in medically similar circumstances do not have equal access to services. As a result, unnecessary frustration and suffering is caused to those on long waiting lists (Department of Health. 1989, 238).

In response the commission recommended the introduction of 'an objective system of assessment for access to publicly funded hospital services', which would in turn involve the introduction of a single waiting list with admission to care based on 'order of medically established priority' (Department of Health 1989, 235). And the commission envisaged that the medical staff would play a significant role in the development of admission policy for hospitals The need to monitor the balance at aggregate level, between public and private care, was also recognised. Reducing waste in the use of expensive hospital resources would, they also acknowledged, require the more active involvement of clinicians in management.

The roles of the different types of hospitals (hospitals designated as national centres for particular specialities and local general hospitals) would have to be more clearly defined, and some restriction of patient choice would be necessary if expensive hospital services were to be deployed in the most cost effective manner, the commission argued. In this context the commission made a strong case for strengthening the management capacity of the system. While the general management model (unitary management) was proposed, the commission recognised as essential a significant involvement of clinicians in the management process. The use of performance measures, in the commission's view, is the key to reducing uncertainty and improving efficiency and effectiveness. It recognised that the increasing complexity of the management function in health care will in turn require a move towards professionalising management.

In more specific terms, the commission recommended the introduction of activity-based funding for hospitals and acknowledged with approval the Department of Health's work in this regard. Consultants' contracts in the public system, it argued, ought to be more specific with regard to their core responsibilities. The commission also recommended, in view of consultants' freedom to undertake private practice, the introduction of an agreed system of monitoring the public commitment in consultants' contracts (Department of Health, 1989, 274).

Developments in hospital policy since the commission report was published underline the continuing commitment of the Department of Health to making the process of managing hospital resources more transparent and accountable.

Hospital funding is now partly allocated on a case-mix basis and in the process hospital information systems have been upgraded and improved.

THE 1994 HEALTH STRATEGY DOCUMENT

In 1994 the Department of Health published a health strategy document entitled *Shaping a Healthier Future – A Strategy for Effective Healthcare in the 1990*. In that document the Department of Health reiterated its commitment to the principles of equity, quality and accountability. These principles would be translated into practice through the greater use of information, research and evaluation which would help to determine health need and the appropriate responses objectively.

In general, the *Strategy* advocated a shift to an outcome-driven, accountable health service where those providing services would take responsibility for achieving agreed objectives. Need determination would be a much more rational undertaking, with measurement playing a greater part than it had in the past. The quality of care would, it promised, be assessed from both a technical and a client point of view. Overall there is a greater concern with questioning and evaluating the performance of all services, and a commitment to developing an integrated service plan based on objective need assessment. For voluntary hospitals in particular it proposed the development of formal agreements that relate to health plans for their wider catchment areas.

MEDICAL CONSULTANTS' PERSPECTIVES

The period from the mid-eighties has, as the foregoing review of policy development shows, been one of significant change and development in Irish health and hospital policy. Many changes· in hospital management and organisation have been introduced and many more proposed, all reflecting the new emphasis upon managing services in as accountable transparent, efficient and effective a manner as possible. The key to this, according to current policy thinking (reflected in both the *Report of the Commission on Health Funding* and the strategy document) lies in the greater use of measurement, explicit guidelines and protocols, all of which should reduce uncertainty and make it possible to plan and actively manage services within agreed and explicit policy guidelines. Viewed from the implementation level, however, the reality is more complicated. An analysis of hospital consultants' views on the issues highlights the importance of attending to the prevailing organisational context including management and professional cultures, so that implementation strategies go with the institutional grain rather than against it at organisational level.

Below, the results of in-depth interviews with twenty-nine hospital consultants working in the public voluntary hospitals in Dublin are presented and discussed. Consultants' views on various aspects of health policy were explored, as was their understanding of their role within the public system.

CONSULTANTS' CONCEPT OF PUBLIC SERVICE

Few of the consultants interviewed would use the term 'public service' to describe the nature of their work in the public system. Generally they do not identify very much with the Department of Health or with the state, and refer only to the Department of Health's role as paymaster.

At the same time consultants do have a strong concept of 'public service', but their concept of 'public service' is through a different route, based upon a strong identification with their hospital and its history and tradition and upon professional values. Many consultants refer to the role of the medical profession in founding some of the main public voluntary hospitals. Some also refer to the often heroic sacrifices of doctors working within the dispensary and workhouse system. Consultants see the history of the hospital and the profession as intertwined and they value the traditional involvement of Irish doctors in the management of hospitals.

Many consultants used the term 'ethos of care' to describe what it is that forges such strong loyalty to their hospital. This did not refer particularly to a religious ethos as such, but to the fact that Irish hospitals are, in the consultants' view, very 'caring', 'patient-centred' institutions. Here again they saw a merging of medical and hospital values. A minority of consultants did make some negative remarks about hospital tradition and identity. These consultants were referring to the poor law workhouse tradition and the low quality of care provided. They wished to distance the modern hospital as a centre of excellence from its origins in the poor law. Others, who reacted negatively to tradition, referred to 'medical and religious mafias'. The majority of consultants were proud of their hospital's tradition and history. Generally consultants saw themselves working for their hospital rather than for the Department of Health as such. Their identification with their hospital is reinforced by their professional values – for instance the opportunity to practice medicine in a teaching hospital which has an international reputation and a strong medical tradition.

LOYALTY AND INDEPENDENCE

Eight secretary managers were also interviewed, and interestingly they were also primarily motivated by loyalty to the institution rather than to the Department of Health or to the state. They shared consultants' identification with the history of the public voluntary hospitals and valued, as did consultants, some institutional autonomy from the state. Both consultants and hospital managers refer to the freedom voluntary hospitals have to appoint their own consultants, and to the importance of having an independent board in protecting the hospital' s autonomy. Hospital managers were however more aware and supportive of the Department of Health's wider policy brief than the consultants.

Consultants' views on the Department of Health's role also mirror their strong support for the autonomy enjoyed by their hospitals. Overwhelmingly, they regarded some degree of autonomy for their hospital from the Department of Health as highly desirable. Interestingly, consultants in hospitals with Department of Health and Eastern Health Board officials on their board felt that their hospitals enjoyed a significant degree of independence. However, what the majority of consultants feared was an erosion of their independence, their identity and their freedom to innovate and provide a high quality service.

Consultants identified the participation of doctors in decision-making at all levels in hospitals as important in sustaining professional commitment and in fostering good relations between management and clinicians. Several expressed the fear that voluntary hospitals might become like health board hospitals, where they perceived consultants as having little voice in decision-making. In this context consultants saw the independent hospital board as an important feature of the system. Some referred to the role of the board as that of overseeing the functioning of the hospital in the public interest. In this context, they regarded the board's composition as very important.

There were mixed views on the involvement of Department of Health in hospitals. Some consultants, mostly in the independent voluntary hospitals, argued against this on the grounds that it would compromise the independence of the hospitals. However, at least as many from this sector would welcome a Department of Health involvement in the interest of greater accountability. Some consultants made the point that joint board hospitals got relatively more funding because of the Department of Health's representation on their boards, and accordingly argued for the involvement of the Department of Health. All consultants distrusted politicians on boards because they 'do not know the business' or more often, because consultants claim politicians use controversy for political ends and have little loyalty to the hospital itself.

Generally, consultants' primary concern was that their hospitals would continue to provide high quality care and retain their caring ethos and commitment to excellence.

HOSPITAL MANAGEMENT

Overall, consultants rated hospital management very highly. They in fact identified strongly with hospital CEOs and managers. This shared strong loyalty to their hospital provided the common basis for the very good relationship between consultants and managers, confirmed in interviews with eight CEOs. Any tension in the relationship consultants blamed largely on external constraints, mostly lack of resources. The under-resourcing of the system, as they saw it, accounted for too much 'fire fighting', 'crisis management' and lack of long-term planning. Some consultants were critical of the style and type of management in hospitals and argued for more 'rational approaches', 'more transparency'. In their view management is not 'proactive' enough, or lacks the skills or education to manage effectively. Some refer to the lack of efficiency incentives i.e. the opportunity to retain savings.

CONSULTANTS' CONCEPT OF MANAGEMENT

Consultants were asked for their views on the proposed clinical directorates (a formal system of clinical budgeting at unit/speciality level) and on what role consultants might play in management. Consultants' views fell into two main categories: those who favour some form of professional control (about two-thirds) and those who favour lay management (about one-third). The majority of those who favour professional control advocate a partnership/team based approach. Only a minority of this group favoured a strong medical directorate along the lines of the mastership (Irish) or the medical CEO (US) model.

There was considerable diversity in their views on consultants' involvement in management; but all consultants interviewed were concerned that, whatever the model chosen, dialogue and communication should not be replaced by hierarchical control systems. They emphasise the importance of clinical knowledge and its role in improving management decision-making and in legitimating and providing effective management. They also cite the 'public interest' (protecting patients) as a reason for significant professional involvement in management. However, consultants had some concerns about the proposed Clinical Directorate (CDs). 'Who would these CDs be?' was a question many rhetorically asked. Unless the consultant appointed to the post has 'credibility and the confidence of his/her colleagues, clinical directorates would not be effective, they argued. It is essential in their view to appoint someone who is respected professionally and who continues to practice. Alternatively, consultants could be appointed to CD posts for a limited period and then, like the mastership, return to full practice. They were aware of the importance of incentives to attract appropriate and representative consultants.

The question of trust was very important to consultants – some were concerned that appointees to CD posts might be tempted to treat their own speciality more favourably than others.

Generally consultants approved of approaches to management that facilitated the participation of consultants in management. Many refer favourably to the current style of management, which they describe as based on 'negotiation and participation'. In this context consultants refer with approval to the fact that managers and consultants work together in negotiating with the Department of Health. Overall, consultants emphasise the need to develop a model of management that is compatible with the existing organisational and professional culture (a view shared by the managers interviewed).

PRIVATE PRACTICE AND THE PUBLIC SYSTEM

In a public health care system like the Irish one, where hospital consultants' contracts give them considerable freedom to practice private medicine on and off site, the management challenge (at hospital and policy levels) is all the greater. It seemed appropriate to discuss the concerns raised by the Commission on Health Funding, among others, about managing the mix of public-private practice in the public interest.

All except one consultant were in favour of the mix of public and private practice in the public system. Consultants gave a range of reasons for supporting the status quo. A number of consultants cited the Department of Health's support for the mix and claimed that private practice acted as a sort of 'safety valve' for an already overburdened public system. Consultants also suggested that public hospitals are increasingly dependent on VHI revenue. In addition to resources, consultants also cited reasons relating to 'public/patient interests' and professional values (notably their autonomy) for supporting the current situation.

If consultants' private practices are on site, they argue, then the public system benefits from the greater availability of consultants to public patients. They claim that private practice in public hospitals also helps to maintain standards, as it provides a more integrated system where the public patient benefits from the higher expectations and demands that more articulate private patients bring to the institution.

Others defended private practice on the grounds that it gives the professionals a measure of independence and enables them to act as a stronger advocate of the patient within the public system. Private practice was perceived as providing a 'balance' to the power of the Department of Health. Many consultants refer with pride to the strong vocational commitment in Irish medicine which they compare with its erosion, as they see it, in the UK. This vocational commitment is, they say, the quid pro quo for the autonomy they enjoy. It is also desirable, in the public interest, that patients have a choice, and can seek a second opinion outside the state system.

Consultants emphasised the importance of what they refer to as 'the goodwill factor' (which they suggest is plentiful in the Irish context) in supporting high quality care in the public system. In general terms consultants claimed there was little abuse of private practice by consultants; most consultants do more than their contracted hours. In fact they claimed that the competitive ethos inherent in a mixed system creates a flexible motivated dynamic profession. Many cited the involvement of consultants in management committees, fundraising efforts, etc., as evidence of the high commitment of Irish consultants to the public system.

Consultants were not altogether uncritical of private practice. Many recognised the need to oversee and monitor the public/private bed balance. A number of consultants suggested that too much private practice could damage and undermine the public system. It was also acknowledged that in some cases the attractions of private practice have weakened individual consultants' commitments to their public practice. Private practice can weaken the team concept, which is so important in the public system.

The vast majority of consultants claimed they got most of their professional satisfaction from their work in the public system. In spite of the frustrations (overcrowded outpatient departments, bed shortages), many cited the vocational element of caring for socially deprived, sicker patients in the public system as being more challenging and rewarding professionally than private practice.

On the question of motivation, consultants regard their intrinsic motivation as very important. They defined this in terms of 'pride in the job well done', 'recognition from peers', 'excellence' and self esteem'. On this issue most rated their public practice higher than their private practice. The public hospital's history, tradition and identity was, in this context, also very much bound up with professional self-definition and standing.

Practice Plans, DRGs and Bed Management

Consultants considered the likely impact some key aspects of the new management strategies for hospitals would have on their practices. Three specific strategies were reviewed with them, namely practice plans, DRGs and bed management.

Overall, their concern was that the system would become rigid, inflexible or bureaucratic and that they would lose control of important areas of medical decision-making. They also expressed some concern that the new management strategies would initiate a process of deprofessionalisation, or that professional values and their strong identification with their practice and with the hospital would be undermined or weakened. Despite some criticism and reservations, consultants in principle endorsed the current direction of change towards more rational information-based management strategies.

Practice Plans

A practice plan is a plan agreed between a consultant and his/her hospital, specifying the core responsibilities of the consultant post. While consultants had no objection in principle to these, many had concerns about the unintended consequences of their specific applications. The vast majority of consultants were opposed to closely supervised individual practice plans, and many used the term 'clock-watching' to encapsulate their dislike of the idea. They feared the erosion of the trust that exists currently between management and consultants – a trust, they claim, that is accompanied on both sides by a huge commitment and willingness to take responsibility. It is a 'legalistic' interpretation of practice plans that consultants fear. Most favour unit-level plans rather than individual-based plans. Many saw the benefits for their hospital of planning of this type, which they agreed would highlight among other things the need for more and better facilities for consultants.

Diagnosis Related Groups (DRGs)

On the question of DRGs (a case mix system for measuring and funding hospital activity), consultants have a range of views. Generally they felt that hospitals would gain from a DRG system if the information on which it is based is accurate. Some actually were very positive and felt that a DRG system would be fairer and more rational. Many consultants had concerns about the type of information used in the construction of DRGs, feeling that it was biased towards funding activity and might encourage procedure-oriented practice to too great an extent. Physicians were particularly concerned about this. Generally consultants felt that a similar type of investment in information on audit and quality was required in the interest of balancing efficiency and quality concerns.

Bed Management

Most consultants reacted negatively to the concept of bed management. Many made the point that in the context of the bigger problems of bed shortage/casualty overflow, it is difficult to see how a bed management system would work. Most consultants would prefer a unit-based rather than a central system. Many claimed that the bed manager had no real power, but the strength of their reaction to central bed management suggests that consultants have in fact experienced some loss of control and power as a result of the introduction of bed management.

MANAGING CHANGE: SOME KEY ISSUES

The research results outlined above reveal strong medical and management cultures in Irish public voluntary hospitals that are mutually reinforcing. Consultants' identification with their hospitals is an important source of motivation and defines their public service orientation in the Irish context. Strong institutional loyalty on the part of managers and consultants facilitates a strong corporate spirit that in turn provides consultants and managers with a common purpose and an incentive to work together.

Hospital managers' identification with business management role models, and consultants' independent contractor status coupled with the freedom to practise private medicine, reinforce the identification of consultants and managers with their institutions. The management structure of hospitals and the tradition of involvement of the medical professionals in the management of those hospitals at all levels further strengthens consultants' identification with them.

Management-professional relationships in the Irish hospital context are collegiate and are characterised by high levels of trust and mutual support. This strong collegiate culture is a defining characteristic of these hospitals. Management is based upon negotiation and an appeal to organisational and professional values. This culture is of course gradually incorporating new management strategies, structures and techniques in response to a changing external environment. This inevitably challenges the existing management and professional cultures.

Management strategies that are based on measurement, guidelines and protocols are not incompatible with collegiate forms of control, such as that witnessed in Irish public voluntary hospitals. However the successful incorporation of such new strategies (i.e. practice plans, activity based funding etc.) will require appropriate adaptation to the existing professional-management culture.

Increasingly international management literature recognises the importance of attending to the existing cultural context and adapting proposed new management techniques and strategies, so that one 'builds on the prevailing culture thereby winning support for the proposed changes' (Nevis *et al.* 1995; Jacobs 1994; Mayne *et al.* 1992). In fact the degree to which a system might move towards measurement, and in which areas of hospital management, needs to be addressed specifically in each health system, because the appropriate balance between information/measurement-based management and management based on trust will vary according to the dynamics and character of each country's health care system.

COUNTER-CONTROL

A negative consequence of failing to respect the existing culture is counter-control. This is a situation where professionals who are not convinced of the value of some element of change, or generally fear change, decide to 'work the system'. Counter-control is a possibility in all work organisations, but the consequences of the exercise of counter-control are greater in professional organisations where, due to the nature of the work, considerable discretion is exercised, increasing the power professionals have to resist or undermine what they perceive as undesirable change. Reducing or preventing counter-control is an important consideration when significant management and organisational change is contemplated in health care organisations.

CONCLUSIONS

In the Irish context, the consultants and managers interviewed favoured collegiate rather than individual-based applications of new measurement-based management practice. Consultants in particular wished to develop practice plans as group norms. For example, with regard to clinical directorates, consultants wished to retain a collegiate approach by insisting on an appeal to professional (group-based) as opposed to organisational/bureaucratic (individual-based) authority. This is an important aspect of Irish hospital management. Irish hospital consultants were less defensive than, for instance, their UK counterparts (Black and Thompson 1993; Farrar 1993) about the significant use of information/measurement in the management of hospitals – they had much higher trust in management. However they did differentiate between modes of application, and generally their preference was to retain the strong collegiate management-professional framework that already exists as the preferred mode of incorporating more measurement-based approaches to management.

Retaining and supporting the existing strong corporate and professional cultures in Irish hospitals is not incompatible with the notion of delivering services within a national policy framework, and meeting Department of Health goals of providing integrated, co-ordinated health services. Similarly the policy objectives of increasing the responsiveness, accountability and transparency of delivery systems can be met. However, the challenge is necessarily greater in a devolved hospital system that has enjoyed considerable independence. In such a system there is a greater likelihood of conflict emerging between hospitals and wider health system goals, particularly if the organisational or professional cultures or contractual or other practical organisational arrangements unintentionally work against the achievement of wider policy goals. There can and must be some alignment of professional, hospital and Department of Health policy goals. Recent empirical literature on professional service organisations, for instance, shows that an alignment between professional and organisational goals is possible without undermining professional values and identity (Guntz *et al.* 1994; Stevens, 1992).

In more specific terms it could be argued, with substantial supporting evidence from the international health economics literature, that the incentives for private practice (remunerative and contractual) in the Irish hospital system work against important aspects of hospital policy. The financial incentives for consultants to identify with, and commit time to, the public system are in comparison relatively weak. This is not to say that this commitment is lacking. However the balance of incentives for public and private work is an issue that needs to be addressed. Sufficient incentives are needed to attract representative and respected members of the profession into management. The benefits of a mixed system are obvious, but what is at issue here is the need to establish agreed policy at hospital level and at national level regarding the principles that might inform the appropriate management of public and private practice, in the wider public interest.

The hospital board or its governance structure is important in formulating hospital policy. The board has an important role in scanning and perhaps shaping the hospital's policy environment. One way of ensuring a good measure of success is to consider the structure of the board of governance with a view to recruiting appropriate policy experts (as is now the practice in UK Hospital Trusts) who can help the CEO, chairperson of the board, the Medical Council etc. to scan the policy environment and help the board adjust and meet wider policy demands more effectively.

The medical/professional culture is an important influence on hospital governance, and on the overall management of hospitals. It is therefore important that the profession considers how it might at hospital level nurture a stronger awareness and knowledge of Department of Health policy, among consultants. This is compatible with, and need not conflict with, their strong identification with their hospital, its tradition and with professional values. The wider issue of medical socialisation and medical education is relevant here.

Given the increasing importance of management and the need for clinician involvement, it may be necessary in the future for both the Department of Health and the profession to consider how, at undergraduate as well as at post-graduate level, medical education might address policy and management issues.

SUMMARY

The emerging consensus internationally is that improvement in the management capacity of health care systems is necessary if system efficiency and effectiveness are to be addressed. This article is part of this international debate, written from an Irish perspective. While some common concerns have been identified in the international health management literature, it is also recognised that the particular approaches/strategies employed will need to be adapted to work with the grain of the particular cultural and organisational character of each system.

The historical development of a health care system, current policy and organisational context (including organisational professional and management cultures) are acknowledged as important considerations. In the Irish context, as the overview of policy demonstrates, the Irish public (state managed) hospital system had a very poor image up to the 1960s, and until the 1950s did not play as significant a role as the public voluntary hospital system. Despite increasing state responsibility for health care from 1950s, it proved difficult in practice for the Department of Health to effectively co-ordinate and plan hospital services. Between 1960-1980 health expenditure grew rapidly. However from the late 1970s public expenditure was under review and health cuts were introduced. The health cuts, introduced as they were across the board, had a significant impact on the public confidence in the public system and revealed weaknesses in the planning and management capacity of the system. It was evident, as the Report of the Commission on Health Funding was to reveal, that the management capacity in particular of the system needed to be developed and improved, and that more rational information-driven approaches to planning and managing services were required.

At macro level, the case for more rational strategic planning of health services has been made. At organisational (hospital) level, the challenge of the need to shift to more rational approaches is a formidable one. The need to incorporate new management strategies so that one is building on and working with the existing organisational, management and professional cultures is an important consideration. The Irish research cited here identifies strong mutually supportive management and professional cultures at hospital level, both of which are sustained by a powerful identification on the part of hospital consultants and managers with their hospitals' traditions, identities, reputations and autonomy. Strong institutional loyalty is a major strength, as is the strong collegiate professional-management culture. However, there are significant difficulties in regard to aligning wider health policy for hospitals with hospitals practice in a devolved system like the Irish one, where hospitals enjoy considerable autonomy. Retaining this autonomy (which supports high levels of vocational commitment from both managers and professionals) while improving the policy/hospital alignment is the major challenge facing the Irish health care system. In the concluding section of this article, strategies that will forge a stronger relationship between the public voluntary hospitals, their managers and professionals, and national policy are identified.

CHAPTER 15

Financing the Irish Health Services: From Local to Centralised Funding and Beyond

Miriam Wiley

INTRODUCTION

With the establishment of the Department of Health in Ireland in 1947, an extensive range of responsibilities was defined, including the prevention and cure of disease and the treatment and care of those suffering from mental and physical illness. The effective discharge of these functions meant that responsibility for ensuring the resourcing of the health services also had to be vested in this new government department. The evolution of the approach to financing the health services over the past five decades is the subject of this review. It will be apparent that the financing of the health services has, at times, been both reactive to changes in the broader health service system and proactive in the implementation of innovations within this system. This paper begins with an assessment of how a health service which was primarily funded from local sources, when the Department of Health was established, ultimately came to be reliant on the central exchequer for funding purposes. Having traced how the source of funds came to be determined, the approach adopted to resource allocation within the health services will then be addressed. Finally, the development of the health insurance sector within the overall health financing system will be briefly reviewed.

THE EARLY YEARS

Prior to 1947, responsibility for health service provision was vested in the local authorities, and the health services were essentially financed from local rates with limited support from state grants. By 1947, state grants met just 16 per cent of the total cost of health service provision (Hensey, 1959). An extension of state support for health service financing was associated with the establishment of the new government department which was expected to expand the services available to the public. This undertaking was put forward in the 1947 White Paper and given effect in the Health Services (Financial Provisions) Act, 1947. The objective of this legislation was to make provision for the state to pay for the cost increases associated with the expansion of health service provision. The specific mechanism put in place was that for each health authority, the state agreed to meet the full amount of the increase in the cost of service provision up to the level at which state support amounted to twice the level of commitment from local taxation in the year ending March 31, 1948. Subsequently, the cost of funding the health service was to be divided equally between the local rates and the exchequer. This division of responsibility for health service funding had been achieved by the time the provisions of the 1953 Health Act were to become effective. The establishment of the Department of Health and the enactment of the Health Services (Financial Provisions) Act, 1947 were therefore associated with an increase in state support for health service provision at the local level.

The emergence of a debate on the appropriate division of responsibility for health service financing between the state and local authorities is noted in a submission by the Department of Health to the Dáil Select Committee on the Health Services in May 1962. In recognising that the expansion of the health services since 1947 was largely financed by the state, it was stated that this 'was not intended to alter the traditional framework of a service which has always been and still is strictly local in character and which is financed and administered primarily by local bodies under the general direction and supervision of the central authority' (p. 64). In this memorandum, the Department of Health estimated that when the state contribution to health service financing was combined with the contribution from the Agricultural Grant, the central exchequer was actually bearing close to 65% of health service costs compared with a contribution of 35% from the local rates. It was clearly recognised in this memorandum that any decision to shift the majority of the health service cost burden away from the local authority on to the central exchequer would have to be considered in association with changes in the administration of the services. The Department's perspective, at the time, on the relationship between health service financing and adminstration is very effectively summarised as follows:

> In the provision of health services, there is very considerable scope for extravagance and unless the authority which is responsible for day-to-day decisions in the operation of the services is governed by the sense of financial responsibility which arises from having to contribute a considerable part of the rise in expenditure which might result from its actions,

then there is the possibility that expenditure might rise unnecessarily and wastefully *(Dáil Select Committee on the Health Services,* 1962, 67).

THE 1966 WHITE PAPER

The division of responsibility for health service financing between the state and the local authorities was subsequently the subject of a detailed review in the White Paper on *The Health Services and their Further Development,* published in 1966. This White Paper presented a framework for substantial reform and expansion of the health service system and recognised the substantial demands that such reform would make on the financing of the health services. In so doing, the government acknowledged that 'the local rates are not a form of taxation suitable for collecting additional money on this scale' and it was proposed that 'the cost of the further extensions of the services should not be met in any proportion by the local rates' (p. 59). One reason put forward for this decision was the inequity which could result from the variation in health rates between different local authorities, reflecting local differences in the capacity to develop the health services as proposed. Political opposition to financing health services from the local rates had also begun to grow, as the health services were accounting for an increasingly large proportion of local authority expenditure (Barrington, 1987). It was therefore proposed that the contribution from the local rates to the health services would be fixed at the level prevailing in the base year 1965-66, and the additional cost of any expansion of this service would be met by the state. While there were difficulties in maintaining this commitment in subsequent years, annual discretionary grants from the Exchequer helped to alleviate the demands on the rates (Barrington, 1987).

Given the recognised inter-relationship between financing and administration, the government concluded that as the health services would be expected to draw an increasing proportion of the required resources from central sources, a new administrative framework combining national and local interests would also be required. As the Minister for Health's responsibility to the general taxpayer increased as funding from the central exchequer was expanded, so also did the accountability of the minister. The government therefore proposed that legislation should be introduced to transfer the administration of the health services from the existing local authorities to newly enacted regional health boards. These boards were to represent a partnership between local and central government and the vocational organisations, taking over responsibility for the hospital service, the general medical service and the community health services. This proposal was subsequently given effect in the Health Act, 1970.

THE HEALTH ACT, 1970 AND BEYOND

Following the Health Act, 1970, eight regional health boards took over responsibility for service provision in April 1971. Over this period, the proportion of total expenditure met from the local rates was decreasing and between 1973 and 1976, the local contribution to health service financing was phased out completely. As this source of financing was being eliminated, additional sources were being developed with the introduction of EEC regulations governing liability for the cost of health services for pensioners and the insured, in addition to the enactment of the Health Contributions Act, 1971. This act was introduced at the same time as the abolition of hospital charges for that proportion of the population which had limited eligibility. The contributions which were collected through the Social Welfare stamp were intended as part payment for the services which were being made available without charge to this segment of the population. While a system of flat-rate contributions was introduced when the scheme was initiated, in April 1979 a scheme of pay-related contributions was introduced whereby all income earners were liable, with the exception of those with full eligibility and those in receipt of specific social welfare benefits. Employers were liable for the contributions of those with full eligibility.

One of the most fundamental reviews of health service funding in recent decades was undertaken by the Commission on Health Funding which reported in 1989. This commission was established in 1987 in response to the pressures on public expenditure experienced in the mid- to late-1980s with the objective of examining the financing of health services and making 'recommendations on the extent and sources of the future funding required to provide an equitable, comprehensive and cost-effective public health service and on any changes in administration which seem desirable for that purpose' (p.1).The report of the commission covers a wide range of areas, including health service funding, expenditure and eligibility, together with the relationship between the public and private sectors. A key conclusion of the commission's deliberations was that the solution to the problem of financing the Irish health services did not lie primarily in the system of funding but was closely related to the way in which services were planned, organised and delivered.

Issues raised by the commission with regard to accountability and role definition at the health board level have more recently been addressed in the Health (Amendment) Bill, 1996 which is concerned with the combined objectives of (i) improving financial accountability and expenditure control procedures in health boards; (ii) clarifying the respective roles of the members of health boards and their chief executive officers; and (iii) initiating the process of removing the Department of Health from detailed involvement in operational matters. The commission also made a number of important recommendations concerning the interface between the public and private sectors, in particular that tax relief on private insurance contributions should be phased out. To date, progress towards this objective has involved a reduction in tax relief to the standard rather than the marginal tax rate.

The recommendation by the commission that health service funding should be primarily tax-based continues to be supported. Additional funding sources subsequently introduced include the National Lottery and income from hospital charges. Table 1 provides an overview of how the sources of health service funding have changed since the early 1970s. While exchequer funding for the health services increased from 80.5 per cent in 1973/3 to 94.5 per cent in 1977, by 1996 the contribution from this source had dropped to 82.4 per cent. As a proportion of total health expenditure, however, the public component has dropped from a level of 85 per cent in the 1980s to just 75 per cent in the mid-1990s. The growth in the private sector over this period accounts for the 25 per cent of total health expenditure now credited to such sources as health insurance companies and household expenditure on general practitioner visits, pharmaceuticals and private hospital stays.

RESOURCE AVAILABILITY

To facilitate some insight into changes in the level of health expenditure over time, Table 2 shows the percentage change in health expenditure as a proportion of GNP for the five decades since the establishment of the Department of Health in 1947. Up to the most recent decade, the general trend in evidence is an increase in the proportion of GNP devoted to health care. The level of the increase can be seen to vary. The first decade of the Department of Health's existence was associated with the greatest increase in health expenditure as a percentage of GNP, but for each of the four decades between 1947 and 1986 the proportion of GNP devoted to health expenditure increased by over 30 per cent. For the most recent decade, however, there is a dramatic reversal of this trend, with the proportion of GNP devoted to health expenditure being reduced by 6.8 per cent over the 1987-96 period.

A different picture emerges if, instead of taking the establishment of the Department of Health as the starting point, calendar decades are assessed. The expansionism of the 1970s is clearly in evidence as the proportion of GNP allocated to health increased by 56.8 per cent, from 4.4 per cent in 1970/71 to 6.9 per cent in 1979. During this period, public spending increased substantially and health service eligibility and availability were also expanded. The 1980s sharply contrasted with the previous decade, however, as a public expenditure crisis and economic recession were associated with a reduction of 16 per cent in the proportion of GNP allocated to health expenditure, from 8.1 per cent in 1980 to 6.8 per cent in 1989. While the 1990s has developed as a period of greater stability in the proportion of GNP devoted to health expenditure, the downward trend has continued, with a 2.6 per cent reduction from 6.97 per cent in 1990 to 6.79 per cent in 1996.

RESOURCE ALLOCATION

Since responsibility for health service funding was transferred to the state, exchequer spending on the health services has been determined in negotiations between the Department of Finance and the Department of Health, which retains responsibility for policy development and overall planning within the health services. Funding for the provision of public health services is provided on the basis of annual budgets to the eight regional health boards. In general, these budgets constitute a global allocation with the health board having responsibility for allocating funding across the three main programmes, i.e. the general hospital programme, the special hospital programme and the community care programme. In making these allocations, the Department may however indicate a level of funding which would be assumed for a particular service such as, for example, the regional hospital within the health board area.

Health board budgets are determined by demographic factors, commitments to service provision, and the general economic guidelines being applied to the operation of the public service as a whole. These guidelines have particular reference to public sector pay levels which generally constitute the largest component of health expenditure. In addition to service delivery agencies, other corporate bodies and registration boards are now supported by the Department of Health. These include such bodies as the Blood Transfusion Service Board, Comhairle na nOspidéal (The Hospital Council) and the Health Research Board.

When the health boards were established in 1971, the voluntary public hospitals which had traditionally been run by religious orders were maintained outside of this structure. The voluntary agencies providing care for the mentally handicapped were also maintained outside of the health board structure. Funding for the voluntary hospitals and the major mental handicap agencies has therefore continued to be negotiated individually with the Department of Health. Following on the recommendations of a number of consultative reports, the Minister for Health in 1996 announced the establishment of a high-level task force to oversee and manage the development of a new health authority in the Eastern Region (Report of the Dublin Hospital Initiative Group, 1991). This authority would be responsible for the funding of all health services in the region, including those provided by the voluntary hospitals. It is expected, however, that full transition to the proposed arrangements would take two to three years. A working group reporting in late 1995 recommended that responsibility for funding the mental handicap agencies should also be transferred from the Department of Health to the health boards. Following discussion between the Federation of Voluntary Bodies, the Department of Health and the health boards, 'a framework for implementation of this recommendation has been agreed. Responsibility for funding the mental handicap agencies is being transferred to two health boards in 1997, with the transfer to other health boards planned for implementation on a phased basis.

In considering the funding of acute hospital services in particular, the Commission on Health Funding recommended that hospitals should receive global budgets for the provision of an agreed service level. The calculation of these budgets should be based on an assessment of the activity level implied by the hospital's agreed role and catchment area, and the case-mix based cost indicated by the level of service provision. In addition, it was suggested that techniques such as Diagnosis Related Groups (DRGs) or other case-mix measures should be used to determine the level of funding required for the service level agreed.

The establishment of the National Case-Mix Project by the Department of Health in 1991 was a partial response to this recommendation, prompted by the recognition that 'the principal problem in promoting equity and clarity in the way the Department of Health funds hospitals lies in the difficulty in measuring hospital workload in a manner that is equally meaningful to both clinician and funder' (Casemix Manual, 1993, 3). Prior to 1991, the Department of Health had supported initiatives aimed at testing the applicability of DRGs as a measure of workload in the acute hospital setting. A report published in 1990 demonstrated that this technique could be successfully applied to Irish hospital discharge data, and the department then proceeded with the development of a system within which hospital workload measured by DRGs could be related to resource allocation for acute hospital services (Wiley and Fetter, 1990).

In 1993, the budgets for the largest acute hospitals for the first time incorporated a case-mix adjustment within the allocation process. The essentials of this case-mix adjustment may be summarised as follows: hospitals are stratified according to teaching or non-teaching status; activity data from the relevant hospitals are assigned to DRGs and a case-mix adjusted cost is estimated for the individual hospital and hospital group; a budget allocation rate is then determined on the basis of a 'blend' of the hospital's case-mix adjusted case cost and that estimated for the relevant hospital group (Wiley, 1995).

The 'blending' approach was considered necessary because, while the case-mix adjusted costs estimated for individual hospitals showed considerable variation in relative efficiency, it was recognised that sudden and large reductions in the amount of resources available to a hospital would cause insurmountable difficulties for the operation of the hospital. The application of a blend rate of 95% in the first year meant that 95% of the budget allocation rate for the hospital would be determined on the basis of the hospital's own case-mix adjusted cost, while 5 per cent was determined by the case-mix adjusted cost for the hospital group. The blend rate currently in operation has been modified to a level of 85%. With the application of this adjustment, the most inefficient hospitals receive some financial penalty while the more efficient hospitals receive a financial reward, though the adjustments would have to be considered marginal in the context of the overall hospital budget.

HEALTH INSURANCE

The Voluntary Health Insurance (VHI) Board was established in 1957 as a state-sponsored organisation for the provision of private health insurance in Ireland. This initiative was intended to enable the 15 per cent of the population without entitlement to free public health services to make financial provision for their health service needs, and particularly to insure against the higher costs associated with hospital care. With the exception of a number of small occupation-based schemes, the VHI has operated as a virtual monopoly for the provision of private health insurance since its foundation.

With the passing of the Third Directive on Non-Life Insurance for the European Union, however, the Irish government was required to introduce legislation allowing competition within the private health insurance market. The Health Insurance Act, 1994, which came into effect on 1 July 1994, is the legislative basis for the regulation of the Irish private health insurance market and the introduction of competition within this market. The principal objectives proposed for the introduction of this legislation include the following:

* the maintenance of the current system of community rating, open enrolment, and lifetime cover;

* the provision of a 'level playing field' for health insurers with the minimum regulation possible;

* the development of a regulatory environment which would maximise the incentives for health insurers and health care providers to operate efficiently;

*   the maintenance of the position of private practice within the well-
established public/private mix of the health system as a whole.

In March, 1996 the supporting regulatory framework necessary for the
successful implementation of this legislation was signed and laid before the
Houses of the Oireachtas by the Minister for Health. Community rating, open
enrolment and lifetime cover are now mandatory requirements for all health
insurers operating within the Irish market. Under the 1994 legislation, each
individual will pay the same premium for a given level of health insurance
cover, irrespective of age, sex or health status. Open enrolment means that all
health insurers are required to accept applications for membership from all
individuals aged under 65 and that once enrolled, membership cannot be
terminated or renewal refused. The regulations do, however, provide for
maximum waiting periods in respect of pre-existing medical conditions.

The regulations governing risk equalisation are intended to ensure that,
under a community rated system with open enrolment, no insurer incurs
disproportionately heavy claims because of preferred risk selection by other
insurers in the market. Under this system, an insurer with a higher than average
risk profile will receive a transfer of funds from the system while one with a
lower than average risk profile will pay into the system. While the operation of
the risk equalisation mechanism will only be triggered with the development
of serious competition in the market, all insurers are now required to return
data in a specified format on a quarterly basis.

Currently, BUPA is the only major international health care company to
announce its intention to offer health insurance on the Irish market. The
announcement in April 1996 indicated that through the establishment of a new
health care company, BUPA Ireland Ltd., BUPA would be the first company to
offer Irish consumers an alternative to VHI. While there are suggestions that
other companies may also enter the market, these have not yet materialised.

CONCLUSION

When reflecting on the historical evolution of the financing of the Irish health
service, the following comment by Hensey (1959) is worthy of note: 'In the
absence of new or extended services, the percentage of the gross national
product spent by public authorities on health services will tend to fall in future'
(p. 47). This statement was made against the background of a fall in the
proportion of GNP devoted to health, from a high of 2.92 per cent in 1956 to
2.74 per cent in 1958. Hensey was reflecting a view, generally held
internationally at the time, that the need for health care in the community could
somehow be contained and addressed if the 'appropriate' level of resources

could be dedicated to the problem. This view would have contributed to the expansion of state involvement in health service provision in many countries after the second world war, including the development of the National Health Service in Great Britain in the late 1940s. History has, however, now shown this perspective to be misguided as the demand for the commitment of resources to health care has increased throughout the latter half of the twentieth century, with a corresponding increase in the perceived level of health needs in the community.

The historical review presented here shows how the commitment of state resources to the health services has increased over time to the point where this sector now accounts for one of the largest items of public expenditure. While the exchequer commitment to the health sector has been shown to vary somewhat according to the prevailing economic climate, total expenditure on this sector continues to grow.

The extent to which public health expenditure is intrinsically linked to overall government policy on the economy is clearly indicated in the Department of Health's strategy document, *Shaping a Healthier Future* (1994). To an extent, this document builds on, and develops, a number of the issues addressed by the earlier strategy document *Health – The Wider Dimensions* (1986) and the Commission on Health Funding (1989). In particular, a reorientation of the health service environment in accordance with the principles of equity, quality of service and accountability is proposed. In pursuit of greater accountability, the strategy proposes that mechanisms must be put in place which ensure that those with decision-making powers are adequately accountable to the funders and consumers of the services. This strategic overview is accompanied by a four-year action plan for the period 1994-1997 which is intended to present national objectives for service development on the basis of the principles of the Strategy. In addressing the resource commitment necessary for the implementation of the specified targets, the Department of Health states: 'The Government will aim to provide over the next four years the resources for the development needs identified in the Action Plan which is incorporated in this Strategy, while observing the budgetary policy set out in its Programme for a Partnership Government' (Department of Health, 1994, p.12).

While the Department of Health has now achieved the milestone of being in existence for half a century, any review of the development of the Irish health service environment must recognise that the health system of to-day which originated with the 1970 Health Act has its roots firmly in the White Paper of 1966. The fact that, thirty years later, the vision for the health services proposed in 1966 has achieved maturity must reflect well on the wisdom and farsightedness of the architects of this policy document. The summarisation in the 1966 White Paper of the factors influencing health expenditure, and the likely direction such expenditure would take in the future, continue to hold true to-day and may also be expected to remain valid through to the next millennium:

> The government fully accept that those employed in the health services should benefit from periodic rounds of pay increases, in the same way as others in public employment, and recognise that rises in the cost of the services will follow from this. There are other factors, too, which continually tend to augment the cost of the services, including the increasing complexity of medicine, better standards of staffing, rises in prices of drugs and medical requisites . . . and the increasing cost of maintaining the fabric of institutions and the equipment in them. Therefore if there were to be no further developments or expansion in the health services, health expenditure would continue to inexorably rise (p. 58).

TABLE 1

SOURCE OF FUNDING FOR HEALTH EXPENDITURE:
SELECTED YEARS, 1973/4–1996

Funding Source	1973/4* %	1977* %	1980+ %	1996+ %
Exchequer	80.5	94.5	87.9	8.24
Rates	13.9	—	—	—
Hospitals Sweepstakes	0.6	0.5	—	—
Health Contributions	3.8	4.0	6.4 —	8.7
EU Receipts	1.2	1.0	1.5	2.1
Lottery	—	—	—	0.8
Local Income	—	—	4.2	6.0
Local Income	100	100	100	100

Source: *Hensey, B. (1979)
†Department of Health, 1996.

Table 2

HEALTH EXPENDITURE AS A PROPORTION OF GNP:
CHANGES IN THE FIVE DECADES SINCE 1947*

Health as % of GNP
*The data presented here are intended to show broad changes in trends over
the period and should be treated with caution as approaches to compiling
this series may have changed over time.

Source: Hensey (1959)[1]
Tussing (1985)[2]
Department of Health (1996)[3]

	Beginning of Period % of GNP	End of Period % of GNP	Percentage change in health expenditure as % of GNP
1947[1]–1956[1]	1.7	2.9	7.06
1957[1]–1966/67[2]	2.9	3.8	31
1967/68[2]–1976[2]	3.8	6	57.9
1977[2]–1986[3]	6	7.7	30
1987[3]–1996[3]	7.3	6.8	–6.8

CHAPTER 16

Resolving Conflict in the Health Services: A Staff-side Perspective

Harold O'Sullivan

Before my appointment as General Secretary of the Irish Local Government Officials' Union in May 1964, I had served for fourteen years as a health inspector with Waterford and Louth County Councils. Having previously served in the Defence Forces during the Emergency and subsequently with Bord na Mona and Kildare County Council, I was fortunate to qualify as a health inspector in the last of the 'quickie' courses held for that grade in 1949. I have therefore a close recollection of the emergence of the post-war public health services introduced by the Health Act 1947, and of the general administration of the health services by the county councils until that system of administration was substantially replaced by the Health Act 1970. That earlier period was one of 'lean management', so fashionable today amongst many management consultants, where the county/city manager had executive responsibility for the delivery of the health services within his functional area. He was assisted by the county medical officer and his staff, the county secretary who frequently acted as his deputy, and the county accountant who was responsible for the financial services.

Comprehended ˙within a system of administration presided over by a democratically elected body of local representatives, the services were overseen, managed and delivered conjointly with other local services such as roads, housing, libraries and sanitary services in a manner that still had vestiges of the multi-functional local government system envisaged by the county schemes introduced by the first Dáil Éireann in the period 1919-1921, the twilight years of the British administration in Ireland.

The shock delivered to that administration by the desertion of the Local Government Board by the county councils must have had long-term reverberations within the succeeding system, which in the main assimilated much of the bureaucracy of the old and perhaps some of its prejudices as well.

Successive administrations since the foundations of the state have found it well-nigh impossible to foster and develop a multi-functional system of local administration, at once democratic and autonomous, as if the ghosts of the early nineteen-twenties still haunt the corridors of power in Dublin bewailing the events of their time and warning against giving too much power to local people.

The hiving off of 'technical instruction' and 'agricultural services' into 'local committees' of vocational education and agriculture under the direct control of their parent government departments in Dublin constituted the first break in the system. This development created the precedent that bodies established to deliver services locally should be the legal creature of the parent department, which in time delivered the final coup de grace to the system designed in the revolutionary period by the Health Act 1970. However, in the early stages of implementation of the Health Act 1947, the form and nature of the local administration was of lesser importance than that of getting the new services envisaged by the Act delivered in local areas.

The first part of the period now under review was one of a rapid expansion of the local health services, aided by the provision of a modicum of financial provision from the central exchequer to enable the expansion to take place. The public or preventive health services delivered by the county medical officer and his staff of doctors, health inspectors and public health nurses incrementally increased in numbers, heavily engaged in the fight against tuberculosis and the other major infectious diseases then common in Ireland. They were also involved in the delivery of improvements in child health, notably through the schools medical services, including the provision of inoculation and vaccination services for the prevention of tuberculosis, diphtheria and poliomyelitis. The increased number of health inspectors made it possible to provide more effective services in the field of food hygiene including milk and meat, the better enforcement of public health legislation for local sanitary authorities including the monitoring of water and sewerage services, and housing inspections associated with slum clearance and other re-housing schemes.

Latter day commentators on the decade of the 1950s describe it in bleak terms, as indeed it was for the underprivileged, and I am not aware that things are much better for the same class today. It was however a period of optimism, and as more financial resources became available for the development of the health services, improvements became quite evident in the struggle against tuberculosis and other infectious diseases then rampant but now rare. If political controversy retarded developments in the area of child care, and this is usually highlighted by reference to the Mother and Child Scheme of Dr Noel Browne's day, it is well to reflect on how long it took to replace the Children

Act of 1908 with modern legislation, delayed as much by social attitudes as by vested interests. The primacy of the child's needs was not commonly advocated in the 1970s and 1980s.

INDUSTRIAL RELATIONS IN THE EARLY POST-WAR PERIOD

Although the Minister for Health was the 'appropriate minister' for the determination of the pay and conditions of employment of all those engaged in the delivery of the health services, these were also conditioned to the corpus of law and administrative procedures generally applicable to such local government officials, and for all practical purposes they came under the overall jurisdiction of the county/city manager. Apart from this certainty all other aspects of the personnel function were vague, scattered and uncertain not alone in respect of the all important matter of pay determination, but also in regard to training and other general conditions of employment. The large intake of personnel into local administration generally during the late 1940s and 1950s on rates of pay well below par, even when compared with the civil service, with none or very poor prospects of promotion, or even in-service training, created an industrial relations situation that slowly came to the boil and was to spill over into the 1960s. The stiff-necked arrogance displayed by a number of government ministers of the period to the reasonable demands of staff for parity of treatment contributed nothing positive to the situation, but stiffened the resolve of local government staffs generally. This was to be displayed in the militancy of the late 1950s and early 1960s. If ministerial lessons were learned from that period surely it must have been that saying nothing is best when nothing good can be said and that ministerial interference in industrial relations can often be counter-productive.

Apart from ministerial and governmental attitudes, the negotiation procedures were both complex and tedious and rarely decisive. The County Management Act had given the manager total control over staff to the point where, unless he agreed, nothing could be agreed. Many managers resisted any interference in the discharge of their management functions whether by staff, council or even department, and not a few felt that a corporate view given by their Association had but limited value. Many were paternalistic in their attitudes and 'toadyism' was frequently suspected at the middle management levels. The legislation of the mid-1950s which required the manager to submit for council approval all proposals for pay increases or alterations in the numbers to be recruited muddied the waters still further, putting another hurdle in the way of getting sanction for a managerial proposal, or even for a general pay round increase already determined at the national level.

Further developments in the health services ushered in by the Health Act 1953 imposed additional work on the local health authorities, with consequent increased expenditures. This raised the profile of the Minister for Health as a major player in the activities of local authorities, an area heretofore dominated by the Minister for Local Government, and raised the probability of 'turf wars' between these as to the future direction of local government organisation. In many respects it was to become a struggle between the 'conservatives' in Local Government and the 'radicals' in Health, reflected by the latter in the proto-regionalisation of the health services by the Health Authorities Act 1960. This introduced unified health authorities into the Dublin, Cork, Limerick and Waterford areas. While characterised at the time as 'joint bodies' within the existing local government system, their respective size and the extent of the functional areas served were to provide a pilot scheme which ultimately led to the regional health boards of the 1970s.

Whether the policy-makers in Local Government were alive to the implications of this development or not cannot be stated, but the departmental officials working closer to the coal-face probably were. Local Government was however to be burdened at this time by the half-baked ideas of political parties and, for want of a better way of putting it, strong-willed ministers whose only idea of local government organisation they were prepared to entertain was their own. The commendable though belated recommendations in the Green Paper on Local Government Organisation of 1971 sought to retain the county as the basic unit of local government while envisaging joint working at regional levels where appropriate. Political attitudes retarded necessary reforms at critical times, leading to the final undermining of the system by the abolition of rates on lands and dwellings in the electioneerings of the 1970s.

NEW NEGOTIATING PROCEDURES

The long-running dispute regarding negotiating procedures came to a head when in 1961 the Irish Local Government Officials Union, heretofore a conservative and non-militant trade union, established a strike fund. Shortly afterwards clerical staff employed by Dublin Corporation instituted a 'work to rule' in pursuit of a salary revision claim. Notice had at last been served that the continuance of arbitrary policies would be met by policies of confrontation by the union. Fortunately by this time the managers had become a more cohesive and coherent body capable of a corporate view of local government needs and concerns, matched by a corps of officials in the two departments who were aware of the need for reform. Out of this conjunction of militancy on the part of the union and a management more aware of the needs of the day came the Local Government Scheme of Conciliation and Arbitration of 1962.

Modelled on the civil service scheme, this was to provide a means for the settlement of disputes in regard to pay for several succeeding decades, although it is currently in limbo. Its introduction was accompanied by a drive by such 'professional' bodies as Cumann na n-Innealteóirí, the Irish Medical Association and the Irish Nurses' Organisation, seeking a separate scheme for themselves on the elitist grounds that the negotiation of pay claims by 'professionals' should not be comprehended within a common scheme. The attempt failed, the trade unions making it plain that if professionalism was to be a criterion then their members had as good a claim as any. It was about this time also that a doctors' trade union was formed, The Medical Union, which became a founding member of the Conciliation and Arbitration Scheme. Its establishment was forced upon the doctors because of difficulties they had in negotiating with the Minister for Health, Sean McEntee, a man who was no supporter of the trade union movement.

The 1960s was a period during which pay levels in the local government services increased dramatically, affecting all the categories employed in the health services. Morale improved and confidence was increased not alone within the union itself but also in the relations between union leaders and their opposite numbers at departmental and managerial levels. Inter-union co-operation at the staff panel level of the scheme of conciliation and arbitration was further facilitated by the establishment of the public services committee of the Irish Congress of Trade Unions, making even more effective the voice of the 'staff side' . The establishment of the Local Government Staff Negotiations Board in 1971 was to be a major reform for the management side in that it provided them with the necessary research and other facilities to enable them to deal with complex industrial relations issues at the national level in a more professional manner. The general increase in morale throughout the local government service during the 1960s, together with the mutual trust and confidence developed during this period between the respective sides, were great facilitators in the upheavals in organisation and management of the health services that were to take place in the decade which followed.

BREAKING THE LINK WITH LOCAL AUTHORITIES

There has always been a tendency in the state bureaucracy to believe that the division of government functions between the several departments can and should be readily replicated at local level by bodies or boards owing allegiance only to the parent department. However elegant the division of governmental functions might appear at the national level, and political expediency will frequently add its own distortions, the only effect of projecting that division locally is the proliferation of ad hoc bodies lacking in cohesion and community participation. The continuance of the county and county borough councils as multi-functional elective local bodies, bringing all local government activities within their democratic mandate, never recommended itself to the state bureaucracy, probably because they perceived such bodies as being outside their total control. This may have been why, in the late 1960s, the Department of Health determined to break the link with the local authorities by the establishment of the health board system of administration envisaged in a White Paper published in 1966. While acknowledging the risk 'that the transfer from them of their health functions would so diminish the scope of the local authorities' work that they would become ineffectual bodies evoking little interest in the community', the White Paper boldly averred 'this danger is not real' , overlooking the fact that the issue was not the status of local government but the better delivery of local services within a democratic system based on the local community.

With the appointment of Erskine Childers as Minister for Health in 1969, the necessary impetus was given for the implementation of the White Paper proposals of 1966. This led in turn to several encounters between the Irish Local Government Officials' Union and the minister, the former broadly arguing for the continuance of the existing arrangements and the latter making it plain that even if he were to agree with the submissions by the union, which he would not, he was bound by the proposals in the White Paper. The union argued strenuously that there was no justification for taking general health administration and the community care services away from the county councils, that these were being conducted in a coherent and competent manner by the latter, and that regionalisation would present administrative and organisational problems, especially in regard to the environmental health services. Acknowledging that problems might exist in regard to the management of the hospital services, then as now partly state and partly private, the union argued that these could be addressed by the establishment of three or so hospital boards with a specific mandate to secure a better management regime in these areas. The union also made it plain that if in time the proposed regional health board system was to be denounced as a monstrous money-consuming bureaucracy, then neither the union nor its members working the health services would accept any responsibility for it and would instead place the blame upon its progenitors.

Realising that continued opposition to the establishment of the health boards was futile, and with its prime purpose of furthering the interests of its membership in mind, the union engaged in a complex of negotiations involving the minister, his departmental officials and, in time, a company of management consultants who functioned sometimes as a referee between the parties. What ensued was a consultative/negotiating process between the Union and the Department of Health, out of which evolved the present health boards organisation, its administrative procedures and management structures. Among these was a personnel policy in which the conditions of service of health staffs were to be the same as those applicable in the local government service generally. This avoided the erection of an administrative barrier between the two services and facilitated the mobility of staffs between the two. A comprehensive job evaluation and grading scheme was introduced for the clerical and administrative grades employed in the local authorities and the health boards, and in time spread to other non-civil service areas such as the vocational education committees, regional technical colleges and the Dublin Institute of Technology. A problem in regard to the management of the community care services remained unresolved affecting, inter alia, social workers and environmental health officers; the side effects may have remained to this day. The minister insisted upon an arrangement whereby only a medical doctor could be appointed as director of community care, a concept bitterly opposed by the social workers whose profession, in its origins and in its practice, owes nothing to the medical profession.

The successful transition from local health authorities to regional health boards in the 1970s was accomplished, as has already been suggested, because of the high level of morale then obtaining in the local government service and the existence of a mutual trust and confidence developed between the respective sides, management and staff. The departmental officials involved, while anxious to get on with their plans and to secure their objectives, nevertheless developed a genuine consultative process not heretofore experienced by the union, in which the views of the latter were given due weight. The consultative process involved not alone the immediate union leadership but also, through joint consultative conferences, large numbers from the union membership directly involved. In the management of the transition the key role of Jerry O'Dwyer of the Department of Health must be acknowledged.

Despite shortcomings inherent in its organisation and management structures, the health board system has worked reasonably well. The fact that serious problems still exist in relation to the management of the hospitals services can hardly be attributed to the health boards, because a large segment of the hospitals are private and are outside the control of the boards. The management 'freedom to manage' originally envisaged by the management consultants hardly flowered, not because of any ill intent on the part of the department but rather because of the inability of the public service to devise an adequate system of decentralisation of powers to executive bodies, and of accountability by the latter in the event of failure. This is a problem which exists across the public service and is not attributable solely to health board administration. It is easier to identify the problem than to devise a cure.

CURRENT MANAGEMENT PROBLEMS AND DIFFICULTIES

Despite the old saying, history does not repeat itself, but unless one has some knowledge of the mistakes of the past these are liable to be repeated. The problems confronting the management of the health services are now even more daunting than any experienced in the past fifty years. The evident existence of financial constraints, over the past decade in particular, has made the management of the health services more difficult. With a gradually aging population these constraints will grow more fraught as competing priorities further diminish the proportions available for the health services out of the national exchequer. This reality cannot be ignored. However in the absence of a consensus by all of the existence of the problem, there is a real possibility that the quality of our health services will diminish while the din of political and other controversies rages to no good purpose. The failure to solve the problem of management in our hospital services is perhaps the most striking aspect of the past fifty years of the health services.

While skills at all levels of activity, including medical, nursing and other specialities, have increased and are now more advanced than even twenty years ago, this has been accompanied by even higher degrees of specialisation, using more advanced technological aids, expensive to provide, use and maintain. The concern for patient care often transcends considerations of cost even in situations where cost must be taken into account. Ethical and other considerations make decision making in these areas difficult if not impossible. Yet the financial resources available to hospitals are themselves finite, requiring a degree of prioritising if budgetary control is to have any meaning. But for as long as budgetary control is seen as an administrative responsibility only, it can have no meaning within a hospital where the vast bulk of the decision-making lies with the professionals. Some practical means must be found to bring hospital consultants, in particular, into the corporate management of the hospital services with a direct input at the executive management level.

The nursing grade is a key grade in the management of hospitals, a fact not always recognised even by themselves, caught up in the day to day activities of patient care. Yet at ward sister level and above, their role is managerial both as regards staff supervision and the economic usage of resources in accordance with the requirements of the hospital. Nurses too have increased their levels of skills and specialisations, yet the sheer weight of their numbers and their influence on the staffing and pay structures of other grades make the provision of an adequate pay and grading structure difficult to provide for them. Just as it can be successfully argued that many medical procedures can be adequately administered by nurses, many activities currently within the remit of nurses can be discharged by others not necessarily as well qualified but nonetheless sufficiently qualified for the work to be done. The transfer of such work to non-nursing grades would seem to be a first step in a root and branch review of the role of the hospital nursing service, resulting in a reduction in the numbers employed as nurses while ensuring a pay and grading structure specific to nurses and commensurate with the duties and responsibilities discharged.

While the quality of the medical care given in Irish hospitals stands comparison with the best international standards, continued advances in medicine demand an ever-increasing requirement to maintain and increase standards, not alone in the treatment and care of patients but also in the quality of the management provided. The development of quality management hospital systems which has made such rapid advances in other countries has yet to take firm root in Ireland. Quality assurance schemes are now widely in use in industry, including service industries, providing assurances to the customer that the supplier has taken care that best practices are in place by him in the production of the goods and services supplied. There is no good reason why such a management approach cannot be introduced into hospitals. Total quality management would require a full integration of the administrative and management procedures of the hospital, with the consequent participation of all staffs in its development and future delivery. It may be a hard discipline for managers to undertake, but can hospitals afford not to take radical measures in hospital management to ensure optimal standards in patient care while at the same time ensuring full value for the money spent? Such objectives would also require a full commitment from all levels of staffs who have in the final analysis a common interest in the continued success of the hospital.

Progress in the development of the health services over the past fifty years has varied with the degree of political will displayed at critical times. Vested interests, and there are many of these, exercise an influence far beyond what the public interest should allow. It is little recalled today that the pioneering provisions of the Health Act 1947 were the product of years of intense work, against much opposition, by Dr Con Ward and his staff on the health side of the then joint Department of Local Government and Public Health of which he was Parliamentary Secretary. Before he was able to bring his efforts to a successful conclusion he was brought down by political in-fighting that reflected little credit on his opponents. Dr Noel Browne, the second of the full ministers for health, however controversial his methods, foundered on the lack of support of his governmental colleagues and in particular his fellow party member Seán MacBride, who wilted in the face of opposition from the Catholic hierarchy and the Irish Medical Association to regulations in respect of the care of mothers and children already provided for by the Health Act 1947. The failure of successive ministers to give effect to the controversial Fitzgerald Report on hospitals represents another failure of political will and perhaps illustrates the difficulties involved in securing reform in the face of vested interests and social conservatism. Erskine Childers was fortunate to have had the political consensus represented by the White Paper of 1966 as a backstop. He was however resolute in pursuing his objectives and by his affable manner won over many to his side. Like all his predecessors he was fortunate in the quality of the officials who supported him in his endeavours.

Political decision-making in respect of the health services is not any less difficult today and if progress is to be made, recognition of the need for consensus must be acknowledged by the various interests involved, while they must also accept that final decision-making in this democracy must rest with the Oireachtas.

CHAPTER 17

A Healthy Voluntary Sector: Rhetoric or Reality?

Pauline Faughnan

INTRODUCTION

The history of the health services, in their widest sense, is also an account of the growth, development and changing role of the voluntary sector in Irish society. In the fifty years since the establishment of the Department of Health, one of the most enduring and distinctive characteristics of the Irish health system has been the central role played by the voluntary sector in its operation and development. During these decades the voluntary sector carved out and sustained what are in effect major platforms in the health infrastructure as evidenced in the voluntary hospitals, services for elderly people, services for people with disabilities and the field of residential child care. Equally important, the depth and scale of its contribution is also evident in the 'scaffolding', in the interrelationships between the fragile systems which support and link health platforms. As well as mirroring the legacy of voluntary activity in Ireland, the health field also crystallises in a startlingly concentrated manner the extent of the rhetoric associated with it, and the contradictions and inconsistencies which this masks.

The pace of change in Irish society and the interplay of economic, social and cultural trends have resulted in a radically different environment for the voluntary sector from that of even twenty-five years ago. There is persistent poverty and rising long term unemployment despite the flourishing 'emerald tiger' economy. There are increases in indicators of exclusion and social malaise such as drug, alcohol abuse, homelessness and crime, leading to a demand for new and expanded services. The emphasis on a broader definition of health accentuates the role of social support networks and self-help in relation to preserving and supporting health. Demographic changes such as the ageing population, increase of lone parenthood, migration, and the rise in the proportion of women in the labour market are manifested in the changing social profile and policy concerns. The emergence of ideologies of both right and left promoting concepts such as consumerism and empowerment, and social movements around the rights of people with disabilities, travellers, children and elders are also part of the complex interplay of influences (Gaskin *et al.*, 1995).

The range and complexity of services provided under the aegis of health are very much greater than even a decade ago. There are also indications of clearer strategic directions; the reshaping of health services to ensure that goals, including consumer satisfaction, are met; and a reorientation towards a health promotion approach rather than simply curing illness. Within the voluntary sector itself fundamental changes are evident. The predominance of religious and philanthropic bodies has given way to a much more diverse and broadly-based involvement; bodies with a social change agenda contrast with those concerned strictly with filling the gaps; the tradition solidly grounded in charity and paternalism is paralleled by movements emanating from social solidarity and civil rights. These dimensions are all part of the legacy inherited as we move towards the twenty-first century and each is still discernible to varying degrees in the voluntary sector as manifested in Irish society.

It is a diverse and complex sector which lacks clear boundaries. It is also a sector about which there is little systematic information and where there is remarkably little regulation. Even the exact number of active organisations is not known, as there is no national system of registration. Attention is frequently drawn to differences between the welfare oriented voluntary sector and a distinct community sector. In many respects the term 'voluntary' is misleading; 'third sector' is probably a more accurate description. Whether referred to as third sector, voluntary, or voluntary and community the sector encompasses a multitude of different types, varying levels of organisational formality, powered by differing visions and goals and resourced in human terms by various combinations including paid staff, volunteers, unpaid workers and religious personnel. This sector has played a major role within the health services in Ireland since long before the establishment of the Department of Health. While the nature of this role has changed very significantly it has and continues to be a strong and enduring feature of the Irish social landscape. This is quite different from the situation in the UK, where Billis describes the sector, like some remote tribe, as being 'discovered' or more accurately 'rediscovered' in recent years (Billis, 1992).

The institutional legacy which had such an enormous influence on health policy in this country cannot be separated from the role played by the voluntary sector, and in particular the religious orders. The involvement of religious orders in voluntary hospitals and residential care gave the church an important place in the organisation of the health services (Barrington, 1987).

As the focus moved from the large-scale institution to alternative forms of residential provision to community care, and the county no longer formed the unit of administration, voluntary organisations continued to reside at the core of the growing health services. In the current decade the *Health Strategy*, with its principles of equity, quality of service and accountability, acknowledges the integral role which the voluntary sector plays in the provision of health and personal social services in Ireland, a role which it suggests is unparalleled in any other country. One of the many strengths of the health system which the *Strategy* identifies is the 'strong voluntary sector which provides an integral part of the public system without foregoing the benefits of independence and flexibility' (*Shaping a Healthier Future,* 9).

While discussions in Ireland on the voluntary sector have been awash with rhetoric for decades and its importance and contribution repeatedly acclaimed, there is a serious dearth of evidence in our institutional development to support it. The challenge in the closing years of the millennium is to move beyond the rhetoric, to evolve the structures required for the voluntary sector to sustain itself and to develop its potential to contribute to a democratic, pluralist and equitable society. This is not a challenge for the health arena particularly nor for the statutory sector alone. But the part played by the voluntary sector in Ireland, the value placed on its contribution and the impact of the institutional frameworks on its operation are encapsulated in the health arena. Furthermore, it is encapsulated in the detail rather than in the rhetoric and the generalities. This essay provides an overview of the operation of the voluntary sector since the 1970s when the existing health structures were established. It focuses initially on major characteristics of the sector as manifested in the health arena and then examines the institutional context and framework for voluntary action in Ireland.

CHARACTERISTICS OF VOLUNTARY SECTOR ACTIVITY SINCE THE 1970s

A MAJOR SERVICE PROVIDER

Voluntary organisations in Ireland were often sole providers of health services long after their importance as core-services was recognised by the state. The history of the health services from the 1970s also shows many voluntary organisations to the forefront in developing community-based services at a time when health board services were underdeveloped or nonexistent. Writing in 1980, Curry claimed that despite the improvements in the provision of statutory services, the role of voluntary organisations in the social services field had not diminished and that an upsurge in activity was evident (Curry, 1980). In some spheres the dominant service provider role was maintained by these voluntary organisations. For example, a comprehensive range of services for people with learning disabilities, provided over the decades by a number of large non-governmental organisations, now operates within a framework of a quasi-contract culture with statutory agencies. While the source and method of funding may have changed, such organisations continue to be the major suppliers in a national network of services.

In the early 1980s various bodies such as NESC and the Task Force on the Child Care Services recognised the contribution of the voluntary sector in key areas of provision and pointed to the effectiveness of the services offered. Over the years newly recognised areas of need such as youth homelessness, drug addiction, lone parenting and long-term unemployment emerged, with voluntary organisations frequently charting a path in responding. As the move towards community care gathered momentum, provision by voluntary organisations at national level was paralleled by the development of local structures, focusing initially on the care of elderly persons and subsequently embracing other population groups.

Even in the role of health services provider, a huge diversity emerged within the voluntary sector over the decades. Because the focus of the various organisations tended to be particularistic, their growth resulted in a 'patchy' distribution of services. The unevenness derived not only from the particularistic focus but from the absence of co-ordination, both among voluntary organisations and between the voluntary and statutory sectors. While this situation led to the non-availability of services in some areas and for some groups, it also led to duplication. The poor co-ordination was evident at local community level as well as in national services. In 1981 Kennedy claimed that 'lack of co-ordination was the salient feature of voluntary bodies in most communities' (Kennedy, 1981, 33). The unevenness and the lack of co-ordination have persisted and are clearly inimical to the stated principle of equity which underlies the *Health Strategy*. They also raise the wider question as to the appropriate sphere of action for voluntary agencies and the proper role of the state in the provision of services and in ensuring equity for all citizens. The current *Health Strategy* addresses the structures within which large voluntary organisations will continue to deliver services. However, the issue of appropriate roles of the voluntary and statutory sectors in the provision of basic services has not yet been debated and is critical to the future service-providing role of the voluntary sector.

DEVELOPMENTAL ROLE OF THE VOLUNTARY SECTOR

In addition to providing services, many of them core services, voluntary organisations filled an important developmental function over the decades. Voluntary organisations have 'created' responses, implemented them and developed models based on the experience of their operation and effectiveness. In the process they also shaped health policy and practice in an opportunistic but convincingly grounded manner. Through developing and operating new initiatives, often with financial support from some statutory agency, they were frequently the harbinger of radically new approaches in health care and health promotion. This much-lauded innovatory, pioneering or experimental role of the sector is regularly cited as one of its great strengths and as a rationale for its continuing support.

There is no shortage of areas which reveal this facet of voluntary sector endeavour over the past twenty-five years. Voluntary organisations charted the course from the institution to community-based provision for particular population groups in the 1970s, giving practical expression to the policy commitment to 'community care'. Innovations were evident too in the population groups targeted by the voluntary sector and in the approaches and methods of working with them. Institutional innovation was apparent in new vehicles such as the social service councils, developed to co-ordinate and deliver services locally. However, one of the central dimensions of the developmental role of voluntary agencies is the focus they have provided for multi-sectoral activities:

> . . . because they can often more readily serve the whole person, voluntary agencies are also able to put together what governmental agencies fragmentize through departmentalisation (Kramer, 1981, 260).

It is increasingly recognised that the health remit extends way beyond the Department of Health and its executive agencies and the activities of several other sectors have a direct impact on health. As the Health Strategy formally acknowledges, many of the improvements now sought in relation to health will be achieved by action in these other spheres.

Over the past few decades health and social services were administered by and through different bodies but with little if any interdepartmental or inter-agency communication or planning (NESC, 1995). The National Council for the Elderly pointed out that for various complex reasons we do not have what could be described as an 'ethos of co-ordination' or a climate conducive to bringing about better co-ordination (Browne, 1992). The result of the continuing division of responsibility for children across the Departments of Health, Justice and Education has been described by organisations working in the field as a 'fragmented and incoherent system of residential child care with little strategic planning' (McCarthy *et al.,* 1996, 5).

Voluntary organisations frequently struggled with departmentalisation and centralised planning in putting in place comprehensive programmes which cut across the remit of individual departments in order to be effective and meaningful at an operational level. There are many examples apparent in relation to child care, travellers, youth homelessness, violence against women and the provision of special needs housing by voluntary housing associations. At local community level too, the Lourdes Youth Community Services Project in Dublin's inner city effectively embraced health, education and training dimensions and provided a powerful community-based model of a complex multi-dimensional intervention, addressing a wide range of needs in an integrated manner. In the latter half of the 1980s, retaining funding for those very elements which ensured the integrated and holistic approach presented major difficulties, because they did not fall within the remit of any one government agency.

The voluntary sector also contributed to innovation in health and social services not only by 'doing' but frequently through its important campaigning, advocacy and policy roles. Some organisations such as Threshold and CARE (Campaign for the Care of Deprived Children) embraced campaigning and policy development as their primary roles while other organisations regularly or intermittently adopted a campaigning dimension parallel to ongoing service provision. Allied to the policy remit, yet fulfilling important organisational objectives, voluntary organisations also contributed to policy development through sporadic engagement in programmes of social research.

Of course this developmental role was not universally apparent in voluntary sector activity and where it was it did not necessarily endure over time. The image of voluntary organisations as dynamic, open, responsive and innovative was sustainable only in respect of some. In the mid-1980s, the National Social Service Board (NSSB) concluded that many voluntary organisations quickly become institutionalised, losing the capacity to look critically at themselves and the society within which they work and that, in short, they 'acquire many of the worst features of their statutory counterparts' without having any of their strengths (NSSB, 1982, 7). A decade later, a study on the relationship between the state and voluntary sector confirmed the continued importance of the policy and campaigning roles for large numbers of organisations (Faughnan and Kelleher, 1992, 88).

The contribution which EU funding made to innovation by voluntary bodies in the past twenty years should not be underestimated. The financial support took varying forms: the European Social Fund, which resulted in the major expansion of vocational rehabilitation services for people with disabilities in the 1970s; the broadly-based poverty programmes of the 1980s; the more focused interventions in relation to women and 'the socially disadvantaged' in the NOW and Horizon programmes of the 1990s; or the substantial support through the Structural Funds for local development strategies in addressing long term unemployment and social exclusion in the latter half of the 1990s. European Community programmes provided both the stimulus and the access to financial resources for innovations in service provision, different ways of working and new forms of institutional development. The Maastricht Treaty now provides the first formal opportunity for the development in the Union of a coherent and active public health policy.

While this developmental role in all its varying dimensions may be a hallmark of voluntary sector activity, resources and an infrastructure are required in order to be innovative, to experiment and to critique. Although frequently related to service provision, this dimension of voluntary activity is quite distinct and needs to be nurtured and supported in its own right.

INSTITUTIONAL FRAMEWORK

POLICY FRAMEWORK FOR VOLUNTARY SECTOR ACTIVITY

Despite the importance of the activities of the voluntary sector and the role it has traditionally played in Irish society, there is no policy at national level within which its contribution may be located. There is no clear statement of principles which underlie the relationship between the voluntary and statutory sectors in general. Neither is there agreement as to the relative spheres of competence and legitimacy or the balancing of functions between the voluntary and statutory sectors within the health arena. This is a debate which must take place at an overall level, across all statutory agencies, involving the voluntary sector in all its diversity. There is also a parallel process required within different areas of government responsibility to give expression, in the varying contexts, to any framework agreed.

There have been several abortive attempts by a number of different governments to move towards an overall policy framework. As far back as 1971 a government *White Paper on Local Government Reorganisation* pointed to the potential for local development of voluntary organisations and referred to the need for a partnership between the voluntary and statutory authorities. Hayes recounts how a decade later *The Programme for Government 1981-1986* contained a commitment to a charter for voluntary services which would provide a framework for the relations between statutory and voluntary agencies. This charter did not materialise (Hayes, 1996, 60).

A more recent initiative was taken at a conference jointly organised by the

Department of Social Welfare and the European Commission in 1990. The Minister for Social Welfare gave a commitment to produce a formal charter which would provide a clear statement of the role and importance of voluntary organisations, interrelationships with the state and arrangements for their support. The *Programme for Economic and Social Progress* subsequently committed the government to a White Paper and charter which would set out such a framework and a cohesive strategy for supporting voluntary activity. A Task Force and subsequently an Expert Group were established in 1992 to facilitate the process. Both groups completed their work in 1993 but no White Paper or charter appeared. The subsequent *Programme for Competitiveness and Work* renewed the commitment of the government to a White Paper on a partnership framework. In the closing months of the *Programme for Competitiveness and Work* it was announced that a White Paper would not be forthcoming but that the government had decided to publish a Green Paper instead. The Green Paper was subsequently published but did not become available in time to be covered by this article.

In this most recent initiative, six years, three national agreements and several governments later, a policy framework for voluntary sector activity is still not within the public domain. There is a disconcerting lack of visibility about the complexities of interdepartmental efforts in developing such a framework and whether, and the extent to which, issues of vision, tradition, territoriality or leadership present underlying difficulties.

FORMAL MECHANISMS FOR PARTNERSHIP

Over the years the absence of a policy framework for voluntary sector activity, whether at a general level or in relation to health, was compounded by the sparseness of formal mechanisms whereby voluntary bodies could make an input into policy in relation to their fields of operation. Of course these two elements are inextricably interrelated. As the Combat Poverty Agency emphasised, unless the principles which underlie the relationship between voluntary organisations and the state are clear it is not possible to develop effective structures and mechanisms of support (Meehan, 1992, 7). The past two decades have made abundantly clear the desire of voluntary sector organisations to be involved closely in strategic planning and policy roles and in both economic and social decision-making. Filling that role in a formalised manner has proved exceptionally difficult for voluntary organisations. For a long time the voluntary and community sectors, while seeking partnership with government departments and state agencies, have not been included in policy-making. Existing consultation processes were recently described by the National Economic and Social Forum as limited, reactive and unsatisfactory.

Involvement by the sector was mainly through advisory and information exchange groups which focused on delivery of services. But there were no established structures for the effective integration of voluntary and community organisation into the policy-making process or of articulating the interests of excluded communities (NESF, 1995).

It was originally envisaged that the National Social Service Council (NSSC) would play a major role in relation to voluntary sector activity nationally. As the new health legislation was winding its way on to the statute books, the report of the Committee on the Care of the Aged led to the establishment of the NSSC in 1971. In addition to co-ordinating voluntary and statutory services at local level, the then Minister for Health envisaged the NSSC as providing a focal point for voluntary and statutory services, and the remit of the Council was broad. Over the following two decades it was restructured on several occasions. It was reconstituted in 1981 as the National Social Services Board (NSSB) but only in 1984 was it accorded a statutory basis. In 1988 its functions were once again amended and the terms of reference considerably narrowed. In June 1995 responsibility for the organisation was transferred to the Department of Social Welfare. The NSSB has now identified three major priorities, namely information, social policy, and the provision of support to the voluntary sector (NSSB, 1996). The NSSB certainly fulfilled an important function in relation to social service councils and the development of local information centres and at times stimulated lively debate and critique of the role of voluntary organisations. However, it did not have the scope to fill the broad role envisaged as a focal point for voluntary sector activity nationally.

The difficulties in facilitating voluntary sector organisations to make a policy input were sometimes attributed to a perceived lack of cohesiveness among voluntary organisations. This perception was not without some basis in reality. A fiercely competitive funding environment, combined with an emphasis on the different ideologies and methods of working, provided ample fuel over the years. In Harvey's study voluntary organisations themselves emphasised the under-development and competitiveness of the sector. Many cited the 'independent-mindedness of voluntary organisations and their tendency to guard their territory closely' (Harvey, 1993, 58).

In moving towards a formal commitment to greater partnership, at least at consultative level, a number of changes have taken place at both national and local levels in the past decade which are significant. The Housing Act 1988, the Local Government Act 1991 and the Child Care Act 1991 provide for consultation with voluntary organisations in public planning. The *Health Strategy* also outlined for the first time a statutory framework to be created between new health authorities and voluntary agencies which recognises the role and responsibilities of both parties. Other initiatives were also undertaken at operational levels which brought the voluntary and statutory sectors together in partnership structures to pursue agreed objectives, primarily in relation to poverty programmes, community development and employment creation. The most significant of these, resulting in a new institutional form, is undoubtedly development in relation to area-based partnerships.

In line with the commitment made in the *Programme for Economic and Social Progress,* partnership companies were established in twelve areas of disadvantage around the country in the early 1990s. This marked a very significant change in Ireland in official government strategies for promoting economic and social development (Haase *et al.,* 1996, 2). During the following years, and with substantial support from the EU, local social and economic development was expanded substantially. There are now more than three dozen partnership companies operational around the country, although with assured funding only until 1999. Partnership companies are a totally new institutional vehicle fulfilling policy, implementation and funding functions. The basic rationale of this approach is the creation of a partnership of all key actors – statutory service providers such as FAS and the health boards, the social partners and the community/voluntary sector – in order to combat disadvantage. The partnership model is designed to facilitate a participative process through developing a planned strategy for the geographical area concerned which addresses the multi-dimensional nature of the disadvantage.

FUNDING VOLUNTARY SECTOR ACTIVITY

From the 1970s to the early 1990s, the funding systems within which voluntary organisations operated in the health arena were, with a few notable exceptions, fragmented, insecure and short term. In the current decade new approaches are evident, in both the services provision and community development fields, in relation to contractually based funding arrangements. But the absence of a policy framework for the voluntary sector nationally; the failure to articulate agreed priorities in particular service areas; and the dearth of formal mechanisms whereby a partnership approach, whether consultative or contractual, could be pursued, have contributed to the maintenance of a distinctly ad hoc funding approach overall.

Funding structures mirror and, in turn, reinforce the status of voluntary organisations in Irish society. This is evident in the discretionary basis on which funding is channelled to voluntary organisations. It is evident in the fiscal system with its non-supportive and, at times, hostile tax environment for voluntary organisations. It is evident in the absence of differential funding systems which distinguish between core funding, resourcing of ongoing programmes, supporting new developments and promoting critiques of policy and practice. It is evident in the reluctance of statutory bodies to pay for more than the actual services which come out of the sector. It is evident in the unhealthy dependence of organisations on labour market schemes as a source of core funding. There is certainly a very substantial financial investment made by the state in the services provided by voluntary bodies. The Department of Health estimates that funding voluntary organisations in the field of health and disability alone now runs to almost £200 million per annum (NESC, No. 6, 98). New initiatives are supported and some organisations are well resourced, a proportion receiving one hundred per cent funding. But the considerable evidence available indicates that the framework within which funding occurs is very unsatisfactory from the point of view of the organisations concerned, hinders the development of many and makes a very clear statement about the perceived importance of the contribution of the voluntary sector in Ireland.

A primary culprit is the grant aid under Section 65 (1953 Health Act), the principal funding mechanism whereby health boards support voluntary organisations to deliver necessary services. In 1982 the NSSB pointed out that there was great variation in practice from one area to another in what kinds of voluntary bodies received grants from health boards and made recommendations for rationalisation and clarification. Ten years later a study of voluntary organisations documented a disappointingly similar scenario. In the more recent study, the actual level of funding emerged as much less contentious than its forms, the terms on which it was given and the process required to negotiate it. Extant funding mechanisms were experienced by organisations as uncertain, insecure and sometimes inappropriate and as militating against good management because of delays in payment and their year-to-year basis. The study concluded that there appeared to be no pattern or coherence to funding arrangements with health boards. Historical precedent, access to key decision makers and political expediency were described as providing the foundation on which the funding arrangements between individual organisations and the health boards were initially established and then consolidated (Faughnan and Kelleher, 1992, 19-21).

New service agreements now occupy a central place in the *Health Strategy* proposal for a statutory framework between the new health authorities and service-providing voluntary agencies. The larger voluntary agencies will have service agreements which will link funding to agreed levels of services to be provided by the agency. The *Health Strategy* pointed out that such agencies would continue to have a direct input into the overall development of policy at national level and they will retain their operational autonomy while being fully accountable for public funds received. However, there is no attention given in the *Health Strategy* to the question of funding smaller organisations, or whether under the new health authorities alternative funding mechanisms will be developed. Large organisations providing services for people with learning disabilities and previously funded directly by the Department of Health have been to the fore in examining the proposed new funding arrangements. A Working Group established within the Department of Health recently submitted its report, *Enhancing the Partnership*. The report examines how the principles and commitments outlined in the *Health Strategy* should work in practice for the benefit of the client group, service providers and statutory agencies. It also highlights the implications of the new arrangements for other service providers in the field and particularly those funded through Section 65. The difficulties which current funding arrangements present for these agencies are documented and the report recommends that the opportunities presented by the new framework be utilised to examine the very serious issues affecting this group.

Apart from the movement towards service agreements, two other major developments in the 1990s warrant particular attention, because they have radically affected the funding environment for the voluntary sector. Despite its initial promise the National Lottery has done little to offset the limitations of existing funding mechanisms and locating funding on a more solid and transparent base. When the National Lottery Bill (1986) was passed the focus of who would benefit was almost entirely on voluntary organisations, and during the debate on the legislation it was made quite clear that the lottery money would be additional to whatever the government was already spending.

Harvey's study reveals how the commitment not to use lottery funds for general government purposes was broken almost immediately, and the government diverted the incoming funds into a range of day-to-day spending. The lottery raised substantially more money than anticipated. The intake in 1987 of over one million pounds had grown to more than £265 million by 1995. In the changing priorities over these years, the fields of health and welfare services were major winners. The allocations of lottery money to the Department of Health over a four-year period rose from £6.9 million to £41 million in 1992. While the vast bulk of the health allocation went to ongoing services or to bodies which had a close working relationship with the Department, there was severe criticism from the Dáil Committee of Public Accounts in 1994 in relation to the proportion of the lottery allocation described as 'discretionary'. The Committee of Public Accounts concluded that the procedures whereby lottery funds were disbursed through the Department of Health were not applied in a standard or consistent way and could almost be described as haphazard (Harvey, 1995, 12).

The other significant change within the past decade has been the emergence of the Department of Social Welfare as a key player in funding voluntary sector activity at local community level. The Department of Social Welfare currently provides support for voluntary and community activity through four different programmes, including the Community Development Programme (CDP)[1]. The CDP was set up in 1990 in order to develop a network of community development resource centres or projects in communities affected by high unemployment, poverty and disadvantage. The number of projects increased from fifteen in 1990 to more than fifty in 1995. Projects in the CDP are given a three-year funding commitment. As part of this commitment a programme of work is drawn up and forms the basis for a contract with the Department. In addition to the guarantee of funding for an agreed work programme for three years, there are two other notable features of this programme. One is the parallel resourcing of support agencies to work with the projects on the ground and the other is the systematic identification of priority areas around the country to be targeted for inclusion over the next three years.

WEAK INFRASTRUCTURE FOR VOLUNTEERS

It is essential to distinguish between volunteering and voluntary organisations, although the two are very closely connected within the Irish context. Volunteering as an expression of communal engagement and humanitarian impulses has existed through different political systems and what we understand today as civic society, and is particularly marked in the welfare field (Gaskin and Smith, 1995). The great majority of voluntary organisations in the social welfare field involve volunteers at some level, and the recent large-scale studies on volunteering in Ireland have quantified and documented the nature of volunteering in this country (Ruddle *et al.*, 1995). Irish volunteers make a major contribution to voluntary social welfare organisations, particularly in terms of organisational infrastructure. The most frequently noted benefit of using volunteers is their personal qualities of motivation, enthusiasm and experience. Volunteers are also valued because they enable the organisation to carry out its work through providing a low cost workforce. Large numbers of voluntary organisations deliver at least some of their services through volunteers and many are heavily dependent on volunteers for their very existence. However, there is very little work done in Ireland or elsewhere on the links between volunteer motivation and the quality of the service they provide (Neate, 1996, 5).

There has been a debate in Europe in recent years on the phenomenon of volunteering and the role it should play in society. Much of the recent debate is about the contribution volunteering can make to the provision of services in a pluralistic welfare mix and, for some governments, its potential as a solution to public expenditure and cutbacks (Gaskin and Smith, 1995, 112). If volunteering is expected to play a role in European society as an expression and a building block of civil society and democracy, it must be genuinely open to all. The evidence is not supportive and a clear pattern in the majority of countries links economic status and formal volunteering, with a definite bias towards the higher socio-economic groups. In the Irish study those with third level education were considerably more likely to carry out formal volunteer work than those with primary education only (Ruddle *et al.,* 1995, 61). The reality of the actual costs of 'voluntary' work for people who are unemployed and on low incomes and who are engaged in demanding but unpaid work are well documented in the study of the operation of six community development projects in the Dublin area (Kelleher and Whelan, 1992, 49-50).

Despite the centrality of volunteering, research findings show that supporting volunteers is not a key strategic aim of voluntary social welfare organisations in Ireland. Organisations generally are characterised by the informality of their volunteer management procedures and the low level of support structure for volunteers. Few volunteers get any training for the work they do. A recent study on the training needs of voluntary service-providing organisations showed that while approximately three-quarters made some budgetary provision for staff training, only half made any provision for their volunteers. Yet one in every two of the large number of volunteers involved was directly engaged with consumers in the provision of services (Faughnan and Healy, 1997).

It is apparent that volunteering is not cost-free. If volunteers are to meet the increasing demands being placed on them there must be a concomitant commitment to resourcing the infrastructure of volunteering. There is no such infrastructure for volunteering in Ireland at national level. International research has emphasised the importance of such an infrastructure in order to effectively recruit, support and manage volunteers. Research has also highlighted the potential weaknesses of a system which depends heavily on voluntary provision without offering assistance with management on training (Gaskin and Smith, 1995, 110; Robbins, 1990, 6).

A NEW CONSUMERISM

A consumer orientation has been a stated objective in Irish public health policy now for more than a decade. *Health – The Wider Dimensions* emphasised the importance of mechanisms for active consumer feedback, while the subsequent Hospital Action Plan and reports of the Dublin Hospital Initiative Group reinforced the centrality of consumer satisfaction. The recent *Health*

Strategy firmly places consumers at the centre of its new strategic direction and sets out proposals for their improved involvement in the planning and evaluation of services. The Charter of Rights for Hospital Patients is presented as the first step in setting out the reorientation of one major service and it is expected that further charters will be introduced. At a wider public policy level, the delivery of the highest quality of service by the civil service is addressed in the *Strategic Management Initiative* (1996), which also points towards the use of customer charters as a mechanism for accountability.

These consumer-oriented trends in health and public services in general should not be equated with consumer participation. O'Donovan and Casey convincingly argue how important it is to look at the 'new consumerism' which has generated considerable confusion and ambiguity in social policy discourse (O'Donovan and Casey, 1995). They point out that the term conceals quite different ideologies and interpretations, which range from customer relations approaches, to the provision of information, to consumer participation. In the new consumerism the basic message is that the delivery of public services needs to become more business-like and this can be achieved through the application of private sector principles that are focused on consumer satisfaction. This is radically different from consumer empowerment, where the core concern is with a struggle for participatory democracy by groups traditionally excluded from the policy-making processes.

Nonetheless the era of more explicit consumerism presents challenges for voluntary service-providing organisations and the possibilities of learning from community development methods. The track record of a range of voluntary organisations, as revealed by a study in the early 1990s, is not particularly encouraging. The study revealed that participation by consumers and constituents was evident in many organisations whether in relation to structures or processes, and at both formal and informal levels. Formal mechanisms designed to promote participation ranged from representative democratic structures to proactive staffing policies to providing for structured feedback. While more than three-quarters of the organisations reported that some formal mechanisms to promote participation were in place, the most prevalent were those designed to secure feedback from consumers. Despite this, the study concluded that the issue of participation did not appear to be central in terms of policy or practice except in a small number of organisations (Faughnan and Kelleher, 1992, 107-19).

TOWARDS NEGOTIATED GOVERNANCE

One of the most potentially significant developments in relation to the functioning of the voluntary sector is the change which has taken place in relation to governance in Ireland. There is a movement towards new forms of 'negotiated governance' at national level which impact directly on service provision, on the redistribution of resources and on institutional development. There is evidence of a shift from decisive government determination of public policy, and subsequent bureaucratic implementation, to a more bargained and collaborative approach. The *Programme for National Recovery* in 1987, which marked the start of this shift, was the first of four agreements which by 1997 has brought Ireland to a full decade of negotiated economic and social governance (O'Donnell and O'Reardon, 1996). The PNR and its successors entailed far more than centralised wage bargaining. They involved agreement on a wide range of economic and social policies including tax reform, the evolution of welfare payments, trends in health spending and the commitment to local development.

Voluntary organisations and national networks have long sought representation on NESC, which has played a key role in the national agreements. In recent years the question has been how the model of negotiated governance could be opened up and developed in a concrete way to give groups traditionally outside the negotiating process a voice at the table. NESC itself claimed that the social partnership approach could be deepened and widened without undermining its effectiveness. In 1993 a new institution, the National Economic and Social Forum (NESF), was established by government. It was mandated to contribute to the formation of a national consensus on social and economic matters, on issues such as job creation, long term unemployment, disadvantage, equity and social justice. NESF is a tripartite body which seeks to facilitate a wider participation in democracy by enabling representatives of the 'third strand' to contribute fully to the debate on economic and social policy (NESC, No. 8, 1995).

The third strand represents groups such as the unemployed, women, people with disabilities, youth, elderly people, those who are disadvantaged. It also cuts across the boundaries of what are frequently seen as distinct 'welfare' and 'community' subsectors of voluntary activity. One of the problems confronting the government in establishing NESF was the absence of a structure which adequately represented the voluntary sector overall. Frazer pointed out that in the absence of such a structure in Ireland there are still many significant voluntary groups who do not happen to be part of the umbrella groups and networks represented on the new body (Frazer, 1993, 3). Nonetheless, NESF provides a very important and visible public forum for discussion on key policy issues, allowing new voices to be heard. A key feature of its functioning is the irreducible centrality of developing a consensus on policy options, often in the face of competing interests among members.

At the one time NESF provides both a mechanism for input into national debate and social policy, and an arena within which issues may be explored and consensus secured on how best to meet major challenges in Irish society.

In the negotiations leading to *Partnership 2000,* a new body emerged on the national scene, this time from within the voluntary arena. The Community Platform is an independent initiative by autonomous national networks and organisations combating poverty and exclusion. In the short term, the Community Platform set out to organise the participation of these groups in negotiating a national agreement in a manner that reflected their values, autonomy and diversity. On a longer term basis it seeks to participate in shaping the future of social partnership and to secure full social partnership for the sector at national level. The Community Platform is based on the stated values of participation, a collective focus, solidarity and accountability. Its emergence and the establishment and the outputs of NESF illustrate how the thrust towards social governance has stimulated initiatives which have begun to allow the voice of the voluntary sector to be heard in national social and economic decision making.

INVESTING IN SOCIAL CAPITAL

This overview of the voluntary sector in the health arena over more than two decades highlights both the rapid pace of change of the environment within which it operates, and just how little has changed in a number of key areas. Many of the changes are particularly apparent at community level, whether in relation to community development or local development, where new models of partnership between the voluntary and statutory sectors are emerging. With health strategies in Ireland broadening to explicitly embrace health promotion and concepts such as health gain and social gain, strict distinctions between the various subsectors of voluntary activity are increasingly blurred. The new institutional models which formalise interrelationships both within the voluntary sector and between it and the public sector accentuate just how porous the boundaries are becoming in a number of areas.

Despite the growing interdependencies, the voluntary sector in its various manifestations continues to be a distinctive feature of the Irish landscape. It is also still largely taken for granted. While there is evidence of quite fundamental, if piecemeal, institutional change in some areas, the reality is that there is still neither coherent nor supportive public infrastructures, values or policy-making in relation to the voluntary sector. As Evers suggests, the search is now for policies which do not only 'use' but which help to strengthen. The future guaranteeing and regulatory role of the state in this context is in creating enabling structures and investing in the social capital which is already there (Evers, 1996).

1. Scheme of Grants to Voluntary Organisations/Scheme of Grants to Locally-Based Women's Groups, Men's Groups and Lone Parents' Groups/The Community Development Programme/Money Advice and Budgeting Service.

CHAPTER 18

Strategic Planning in The Irish Health Services

Jerry O'Dwyer

INTRODUCTION

S*haping a Healthier Future*, a strategy for effective health care in the 1990s, was published in May 1994. When the department comes to celebrate its centenary in 2047, it is likely that this strategy statement will be seen as a key event, a major change in official thinking about planning and managing the health services in Ireland. It marked a departure from previous health policy statements in its scope, focus and ambition, and it probably set a standard for strategic statements for many years ahead. It is, therefore, a suitable starting point for reflection about strategic planning in the health services in Ireland.

The publication of the Health Strategy in 1994 was the culmination of a reappraisal of the health services in a wider context which had commenced in 1986 with *Health – the Wider Dimensions*. That review had been sparked off by the twin challenges posed to those responsible for the direction and management of the services – the challenge of achieving the health targets under *Health for All*, the World Health Organisation initiative launched in 1984, and the challenge of managing services with fixed or reducing resources. Between 1986 and 1991, the services had been through an unprecedented period of rationalisation and enhanced productivity, followed by three years of gradual recovery of some of the ground lost between 1987 and 1990. During the decade to 1990, Ireland was one of the very few countries in the OECD to have reduced its expenditure as a proportion of GDP.

Reflecting that unprecedented experience, and influenced by the strategic approach to the planning and management of health services in other countries, *Shaping a Healthier Future* broke with both the content and style of previous major policy statements, such as *Outline of Proposals for the Improvement of the Health Services and their Further Development* (1966). It also set more concrete and ambitious targets for the system as a whole. Although it is still far too early to place it firmly in a historical context, it is perhaps useful at this stage to think of it as marking a definite departure, to reflect on the main new elements which it introduced and to engage in some speculation about the extent to which these elements will be retained and developed in future strategy statements.

CONTINUITY AND CHANGE

Immediately prior to and subsequent to its establishment, the Department of Health has been relatively rich in policy statements. Of necessity and by inclination, it seems that those charged with the responsibility for directing and developing the health services accepted that the path ahead for the whole system should be charted with reasonable regularity and that this should appropriately involve a degree of consultation, before legislative proposals were tabled to the Oireachtas. It is fascinating to observe that the 1947 White Paper was apparently confined to 750 copies; the 1966 White Paper extended to 2,500 copies; but four times that number were printed as a first run of the 1994 document. In addition, an executive summary was provided for every member of staff in the health services and a special video was made as a basis for group presentations to all staff. This concern with extensive communication, with gaining commitment to the way ahead can, of course, be seen to reflect societal and technological changes but it is also an acknowledgement that outcomes which require change in behaviour by all or most people in the system are unlikely to be achieved without their understanding and the support of the majority.

In 1947 and 1966 White Papers were, in their time and context, significant achievements for the politicians and civil servants who promoted them. The 1947 White Paper proposed a very radical change in Irish social policy viz., the gradual extension of eligibility for health services to the entire population. Despite associated controversies, the two White Papers moved the system forward gently but firmly to provide the basis for a significant extension of the state's role and the acceptance of its responsibility to see that the health system achieved certain minimum goals. While their approach to the issue of eligibility for services put the state's philosophy of health care on a new basis, their development of the administrative and executive apparatus was also a fundamental change and of long-term importance. The Health Act, 1970, deriving from the 1966 White Paper, will be remembered primarily for two initiatives: the introduction of the choice of doctor scheme and the establishment of the health boards. The creation of the boards provided the machinery for the rapid development of services and the absorption over the next twenty years of extensive additional functions in the field of personal social services. Despite the importance of the changes and the undoubted awareness among those who formulated the policy of their long-term potential, the language of the White Paper was low-key and reassuring in view of the prevailing alarm among some important interests about the rapidly evolving welfare state. For example, in two short paragraphs dealing with 'general principles', the calming conclusion read:

> The social development of the State, in the government's view, calls for future changes such as are now suggested but the government would emphasise that their proposals do not represent a radical departure from the principles set out in the preceding paragraph.

These principles were, briefly, that the state did not have a duty to provide unconditionally all health services free of cost for everyone, without regard to individual need or circumstances. On the other hand, no service should be designed so that a person must show dire need before he or she could avail of it. The services were designed to meet the essential needs of the population and to maximise the use of available resources by focusing on the specific circumstances of each broad service category, for example prevention, curative, hospital and specialist services.

Contrast this with the content and tone of the 1994 Health Strategy. Here is laid out a firm critique of the strengths and weaknesses of the present system; the underlying principles of equity, quality of service and accountability are installed as the sheet anchor of the strategy; the whole system is to be mobilised to achieve measurable health gain and social gain and reoriented to become genuinely patient-centred; and this is topped off with a four-year action plan, as a first instalment on the implementation of the strategy. One of the primary benefits of having a strategy on which to base the future course of our services is that the system is less likely to be blown off course whenever an unavoidable economic or political gale blows up. We have clearly moved into a new league that is more demanding, and requires a very high degree of professionalism, wherein success promises really worthwhile rewards for the community. In common with both the private and public sectors, the possibilities and challenges are now greater than ever but accomplishment or failure will be obvious to all who wish to interest themselves in the functioning of the health services. There is no longer anything notional about transparency and accountability. The system has offered to be measured on both counts; it cannot complain if the experience is not always pleasant.

Shaping a Healthier Future reflects an acceptance of the benefits to be derived from best practice in strategic planning and management in both public and private sectors. It views the health system as a unity, composed of many diverse parts, which can bind behind a shared vision with increasing effectiveness to achieve significant changes over time. It assumes that management structures, systems and values are now capable of developing and supporting an essential unity of purpose, that the system will function cohesively internally, and that it will relate effectively to other agencies, public and private, whose policies and practices influence health. There is already encouraging evidence of this in the development and implementation of policy in relation to matters such as child care, drugs and food safety.

The strategy is assertively patient-centred. Conceptually, the patient or client is placed at the top of the organisation chart. The scene is set to effect a critical move from concern with the organisation or profession to assuring that the patient or client receives a quality service that is seen as such by both the receiver and the provider. This is a much more fundamental challenge than it might appear, particularly to many working within the health services. Viewed from the outside and from the viewpoint of the prospective patient, there are many aspects of the present organisation of services which facilitate the provider rather than the receiver. It is often still difficult to penetrate the larger units within the services to establish an appropriate relationship with the individual or team who can best help address your problem; the scheduling is usually on the organisation's terms; and there is still a significant problem of communicating with patients and their families. Some of these difficulties undoubtedly arise from pressure on resources and the restrictions imposed by sophisticated technology. The challenge lies in the extent to which deeply entrenched organisational and professional attitudes can be changed to make the service truly patient-centred. This is the touchstone by which the public will judge the success or failure of the strategy.

THE DEPARTMENT'S INTERNAL STRATEGY STATEMENT

The 1994 strategy has been complemented in 1997 by the first *Statement of Strategy for the Department of Health* (recently retitled the Department of Health and Children). The shifts in the department's role outlined in the *Strategy* derive principally from *Shaping a Healthier Future*, which signalled a significant change in direction. The department is now being geared to maintain strategic focus, to know better what is and is not working, and to work in partnership with all the main providers. It must strive continuously for health and social gain, using available resources in an optimum manner.

It is inevitable that the partnership will sometimes be difficult. The department is moving from what might be described as 'co-decision making' with the agencies which it funded to 'measured accountability'. At the same time, it is devoting increased investment to strengthening the planning, measurement and management abilities of the agencies and devolving to the health boards, individually and collectively, a considerable range of functions of an executive and co-ordinating nature. The dialogue about objectives and results will inevitably become more intensive; those who are seen to be succeeding will rightly demand recognition of their achievements; with resources that have to be capped at some level, there must inevitably be losers.

This shift in transparency and accountability will place new strains on the system. Politically and administratively, there is a difficulty in identifying and tackling underperformance; there are always reasons which can be attributed to external factors beyond the control of those who are accountable; in recent years, for example, the focus has been on the alleged inequity of resource distribution, without regard to the reality that resources tend to go to those who present their proposals cogently and with conviction and make good use of what they are given.

It is a serious denial of public service management reality to pretend that the focused application of energy in pursuit of identified priorities does not yield results. It does and it always will, because the competition for public resources is no different from any other – the fittest and the fastest usually prevail! The department and the minister will have to rely on provable objectivity to defend those decisions that temporarily disadvantage agencies and the people they serve; they will have to identify the weakness which led to the loss; and they will have to give their wholehearted support to bringing the losing agency and its management up to the required level of competency and commitment.

THE KEYS TO SUCCESS

The principal changes inherent in strategic thinking in the health area have been touched on in the foregoing paragraphs. If these changes are to be successfully accomplished, what are the requirements and can they be met? The eight requirements which are set out beneath are not, of course, exhaustive but it is hard to imagine success being achieved without most of them being achieved.

The first requirement is that the system maintain its present commitment to strategic thinking and act accordingly. In this, the department has a particularly onerous role but without continuing political acceptance of strategic management as the current best way of achieving political objectives, the best efforts of central administrators and local managers will not achieve an acceptable level of success. In this field, however, one can be hopeful and there is every indication that the health services will continue to enjoy the public service-wide support which comes from the Strategic Management Initiative. Given political commitment, the senior staff in the department must be capable of developing and leading the strategy at national level, and the top management of the agencies must be willing to give of the necessary time and effort to co-operate in that venture.

As in past generations, the greatest health and social gain will necessarily come from prevention and promotion. Prevention will in the main come from the extent to which the environment and our prevailing societal values are supportive of health. In this, the Department of Health and the health system will remain dependent on the policies and actions of other departments, other public agencies and large influencing organisations in the private sector. There is a great deal of work to be done in this area. The Irish civil service is still a long way from being as good as it could be in working inter-departmentally. It is in urgent need of successful working models which will support those who believe that it is possible to achieve major strategic targets that cut across departments and agencies. The department must take the initiative in this and must be prepared to commit a considerable amount of energy to achieving what is necessary in this vital area. A simple first step would be to get agreement that all departmental memoranda seeking government approval would have within them a short paragraph setting out an assessment of the health implications of the policies proposed.

The third requirement for success is that the partnership between the department and the agencies be vibrant and positive. Success must be identified, acknowledged and celebrated and failures seen as the source of learning. The major changes, particularly with regard to the system becoming more patient-centred, must primarily come from within the agencies and from within the professions employed by them. The partnership must be based on mutual respect, on planning that improves with each year's experience and on evaluation that is objective, open and shared. In the immediate future, there is a considerable need for the department to facilitate and support devolution of functions which it has discharged for many years, and for the agencies to become more self-reliant in interpreting policies and protocols which are often referred to the department for clarification and case-by-case decision making.

The fourth requirement is the steady improvement in the ability of the system to measure its outputs and the impact which they are having on health gain and social gain. Apart from methodological difficulties, it is going to require considerable determination and no little ingenuity to devote to this effort the energy and the resources which will be required. We are moving out of an era in which all of the attention has been given to inputs; we have begun the task of measuring outputs; but we are at a very early stage at attempting to look at impact. However, that very process of seeking to measure what may have been previously assumed or ignored, will necessarily change the way in which problems are addressed. We know now, for example, that we are unlikely to achieve our targets in relation to cancer reduction unless we can bring about a significant change in the smoking habits of young people, particularly young women. The very fact of looking at cancer in a strategic way has forced us to acknowledge this at an early stage.

The challenge to measure output and outcome will inevitably focus attention on best practice. If there is one way in which we can achieve better value for money from existing resources through the adoption of one tactic, it is the recognition and application of best practice. However, those who have been involved in seeking to develop and agree protocols based on best practice will know that there are fundamental attitudinal and intellectual issues to be addressed before the majority of practitioners will be influenced in their behaviour by this approach to prevention, treatment and care.

The fifth requirement is the improvement of our ability to manage the complexity of the health services at every level. An activity which has been succinctly described as akin to herding cats, health management is not for the faint-hearted or those who believe that neat models from less complex fields can be readily applied. We seem to have crossed an important intellectual barrier in accepting that we are mainly on our own in devising a system of management that will work for us and will be acceptable to both the practitioners and those who are managed. The establishment of the Office for Health Management is a vital but no more than a first step in what will be a long haul. However, given the very significant improvement in education standards, the high level of attainment and potential of so many people in the services, and the acceptance that management is in need of improvement, I believe that this is an area in which we can be reasonably optimistic, while we cannot relax.

The sixth requirement, additional resources, might be seen by many people as paramount. While additional resources will be necessary and no doubt will be made available, there is no prospect that we can ever reach a situation where there will be anything approaching a match between resources and demand for services. What the strategic approach can help us to do is to make ever better use of existing resources and to base the acquisition and the deployment of additional resources on proven need and anticipated impact. We must also be prepared to allow a proportion of the resources to be used to maintain the system in good working order, whether it be to keep buildings and equipment up to good modern standards or to maintain the managerial and professional fitness of the thousands of staff that are employed within the system.

The seventh requirement is to encourage and support innovation. Within the tighter frameworks which flow from the strategy and its implementation, we must somehow find ways and means of encouraging initiative in thought and action. The present system is not sufficiently supportive of those who want to challenge conventional thinking whether it be a professional or managerial matter, who want to believe and demonstrate that there is a different and better way and who may, in the process, make some mistakes. At clinical level, we have to acknowledge the great deal of uncertainty with which so many professionals are faced in their everyday experience, while seeking to maintain the confidence of the patient or client. It is understandable if we do not wish to add to that uncertainty by introducing elements which are experimental, but that should not preclude innovation based on identified good practice elsewhere or careful assessment of the risks involved in changing the way problems are addressed. Similarly, managers who innovate and look for a new path should be seen as introducing an essential new ingredient into a system that can otherwise become predictable, low energy and producing no better than average performance.

The eighth and final requirement which must be in place is a continuing belief in our collective ability to achieve quantifiable health and social gains through the strategic management of a large and complex system. This is the characteristic which has most markedly shaped current thinking in health strategy. It represents the biggest change from previous thinking and it is a most important counter in the battle against phenomena such as the 'tyranny of the articulate' and 'management by muddling through'. Unless the system is driven by people who have that belief and who have the ability to instil it in those who deliver the services, then the 1994 strategy will not succeed. A system which must be held together for the good of the patient and the community, which is complex and expanding, does of course present major strategic and management problems, but we must accept and overcome the challenge which it poses rather than say that it cannot be done.

HEALTH SERVICES STRATEGY – THE FUTURE

In concluding this short reflection on strategic planning in the Irish health services, it is tempting to speculate about some of the future trends that are likely to characterise strategies in the early part of the next century. The suggestions which are put forward assume that the economy will continue to grow; that there will not be any major ideologically driven change in the way in which services are planned or delivered; and that the mix of public and private provision will remain broadly as at present, with perhaps some growth in the independent private sector extending beyond hospital care into community provision which is now provided almost exclusively through the public sector.

Future strategies are likely to be more influenced than at present by the European Union. The Amsterdam Treaty, assuming that it is confirmed, provides for an enhanced role for the Union in health matters, something which was not expected up to relatively recently and which comes very shortly after the introduction of article 129 of the Maastricht Treaty. The new EU Public Health Strategy for the decade commencing in 2000 is likely, inter alia, to place considerable stress on prevention through making the policies of sectors other than health more health-friendly. It is also likely to give considerable support to the identification and dispersion of good practice in both prevention and treatment. It would be surprising if considerable additional resources were not devoted to further enhancing the safety of medicines and food and bringing the monitoring/measurement of disease patterns to a level which we have not previously experienced anywhere in Europe. We shall also have to take on board the new thinking likely to emerge from the World Health Organisation which is currently up-dating its 'Health for All' Strategy. All these developments will undoubtedly add an extra dimension in the search for excellence and should operate to support positively the objectives of the health service here.

A major challenge to our services will arise from the fact that we have an ageing population and face a likely increase in the extent of cancer, heart disease and dementia. But underlying all developments must be the pursuit of greater equity in health. We shall go a long way in that direction if we can give every child an equal opportunity for good health in the broadest sense of the term. The long-term social and health disadvantages of children growing up in a deprived, poverty-stricken family setting have been very clearly established.

We are likely to see a great deal more attention devoted to inter-departmental and inter-agency working in the pursuit of objectives which are outside the remit of any one department. One can anticipate that, within a few years, probably as part of the next stage of the implementation of strategic management across the public service, there will be a major initiative in organisation development to get over the present difficulties associated with officers from different departments working under the direction of a senior officer from a lead department. Health has a vital interest in the rapid resolution of difficulties in this area. Perhaps more than any other department, the attainment of many of our objectives is outside of our control and we need other policies to be particularly sensitive to their health implications.

Within the health service, we are likely to see considerable attention given to the development, perhaps over a period of up to twenty years, of ever-improving measurements of the impact of services. This development will be supported by considerable systems development which will force and facilitate agencies to communicate better with each other and to communicate better within their own organisations. The numerate aspect of the measurement is likely to be accomplished relatively quickly; what will take a great deal more time is reaching agreement on the development and application of qualitative measures that are real and capable of being administered without greatly increasing the overhead.

Finally, as our inputs become more assured, as the accessibility of services improves, and as we develop our ability to demonstrate good value for money, the challenge of the day will be quality assurance in all its dimensions. Looking back twenty years from now, we will probably have to acknowledge that we are now at a relatively primitive stage in the development and application of quality measures.

The system is appropriately proud of its professional competence and that is a strength to which must be preserved. However, from now on the judgement on the system will be made increasingly by reference to the outcome of various measurements of patient and client satisfaction and of family perception of the way in which their relatives have been treated. There will be additional independent assessment, much of it deriving from statutory committees of the Houses of the Oireachtas and from various Ombudsmen, which will determine whether the health services are achieving the objectives which society requires of them.

Resources will have to be deployed not just to develop new services but to bring to levels acceptable to the users some aspects of our existing services. The tolerance level for long delays in accessing the service, for long delays when people get there, for anything other than appropriate care and respect will reduce steadily, as the economy grows, as more people become better educated, and as awareness of what constitutes good health care becomes widespread in the population. If the health services as presently constituted fail to respond to this challenge, then alternative systems will develop and we will be turned away from what we have been so long creating – the possibility of providing a good, integrated and seamless service to everyone who needs it. The rapidly changing pace of science and technology affects fundamentally the health service and will continue to do so. It is not always appreciated that the system needs to respond much more quickly now than in the past. We can, therefore, expect that the way in which we plan and deliver services will have to continue to change quickly, to find ways of making the large organisation respond as if it were small and flexible, and to absorb the necessary difficulty of constant change without being distracted from the main objectives. The 1994 strategy set the goals of health gain and social gain. These·will have to be achieved while the service to the individual becomes ever more demanding. It is hard to think of a greater challenge to the Irish public service but it is one worthy of the best efforts of everyone who is privileged to work in a service in which so much trust has been placed by successive governments and the public over many years.

References

Akong, R., *Taming the Tiger*, Rider 1994

Barker *et al.*, 'The proper focus of nursing: A critique of the caring ideology', *International Journal of Nursing Studies* 1995, 32 (4): 386–397

Barrington, Ruth, *Health, Medicine and Politics in Ireland 1900–1970*, Dublin 1987

Bateson, G., *Mind and Nature*, Fontana 1985

Beck, A. *et al.*, *Cognitive Therapy and the Emotional Disorders*, London 1991

Becker, G. and Kelleher, C., *Education materials for health professionals on breastfeeding*, commissioned by Health Promotion Unit, Dept. of Health (in preparation)

Billis, D., *Organising Public and Voluntary Agencies*, London 1992

Bisson, J.I. and Deahl, M.D., 'Psychological Debriefing and Prevention of Post-Traumatic Stress', *British Journal of Psychiatry* 1994, 165: 171–720

Black, N. and Thompson, E., 'Obstacles to Medical Audit: British Doctors Speak', *Social Science and Medicine* 1993, 36 (7): 849–856

Bolster, Sr Angela, *Catherine McAuley*, Cork 1982

Boerma Wienke, G.W. *et al.*, *Health Care and General Practice across Europe*, Dutch College of General Practitioners 1993

An Bord Altranais, *Consultative Document on Nurse Education and Training – Interim Report*, Dublin 1991

——, *Future of Nurse Education and Training in Ireland*, Dublin 1994

——, *Supplementary Register for Nurse Tutors*

Bowers, F., *HEP C: Niamh's Story*, Dublin 1997

Bowlby, J., *Attachment and Loss*, London 1973

Bowling, Ann, 'Health Care Rationing. The Public Debate', *British Medical Journal* 1996, 312: 670–4

Breen, R. and Whelan, C., *Social Mobility and Social Class in Ireland*, Dublin 1996

British Medical Association, *Advance statements about medical treatment: code of practice*, London 1995

Browne, M., *Co-ordinating Services for the Elderly at Local Level: Swimming Against the Tide*, National Council for the Elderly, Dublin 1992

Burke, T.P., *Survey of the Workload of Public Health Nurses*, Institute of Community Health Nursing, Dublin 1986

Butler, Sr Katherine, 'Mary Aikenhead 1787–1858', in *Saint Vincent's Hospital Anniversary Yearbook*, Dublin 1984

Busuttil *et al.*, 'Incorporating Psychological Debriefing Techniques within a Brief Group Psychotherapy Programme for the Treatment of Post-Traumatic Stress Disorder', *British Journal of Psychiatry* 1995, 167: 495–502

Byrne, A., 'Nursing has its own Application System', *Irish Times*, 13 January 1997, 4

Canadian Council on Health Services Accreditation, *Standards for Acute Care Organisations*, 1995

——, *Annual Report 1995–96*

Carver, John, *Boards that make a difference*, San Francisco 1990

Commission on Health Services Funding, *Report*, Government Publications Office 1989

Commission on the Status of People with Disabilities, *Report: A Strategy for Equality*, Dublin 1996

Coleman, C., 'The demographic transition in Ireland in an international context' in Goldthorpe, J. and Whelan, C. (eds), *The Development of Industrial Society in Ireland*, Oxford University Press 1992

Commission of Enquiry on Mental Handicap, *Report*, Dublin 1965

Commission on Health Funding, *Report*, Dublin 1989

Commission on the Relief of the Sick and Destitute Poor, *Report*, Dublin 1927

Connolly, J., 'Report on the Inaugural Meeting of the Irish Association of Suicidology', *Medico-Legal Journal of Ireland* 1996, 2 (3): 94–97

Crowley, M., 'The Evolution of the Faculty of Nursing', *Nursing Review*, 1982 (summer): 5–7

Curry, John, *Irish Social Services*, Dublin 1993 (2nd ed.)

Cusack, D. 'Healthcare risk management', *Journal of the Irish Colleges of Physicians and Surgeons* 1994, 23 (3): 176–178

——, 'Hepatitis C – a tragedy in uncharted medico-legal waters', *Medico-Legal Journal of Ireland* 1996, 2 (2): 43

Dáil Select Committee on the Health Services, *Memorandum from the Department of Health Describing the Irish Health Services*, May 1962

Davies, C., *Rewriting Nursing History*, London 1980

Davies, R., *Women and Work*, London 1972

Deloughery, G., *History and Trends of Professional Nursing*, Missouri 1977

Department of Health, *Health Act*, Dublin 1947

——, *Health Act*, Dublin 1953

——, *Commission of Inquiry on Mental Illness*, Dublin 1966

——, *White Paper: The Health Services and Their Further Development*, Dublin 1966

——, *Working Party on Workload of Public Health Nurses*, Dublin 1966

——, *Circular 27/66 on District Nursing Services*, Dublin 1966

——, *Consultative Council on the General Hospital Services – Outline of the Future Hospital System*, Dublin 1968

——, *The Health Act*, Dublin 1970

——, *Working Party on General Nursing Report*, Dublin 1980

——, *The Psychiatric Services: Planning for the Future*, Dublin 1984

——, *Public Health Nursing Services in Ireland*, Discussion Document, Dublin 1986

——, *Health: The Wider Dimensions*, Dublin 1987

——, *The Years Ahead: A Policy for the Elderly*, Dublin 1988

——, *The Commission on Health Funding*, Dublin 1989

——, *Health Statistics 1991*, Dublin 1991

——, *Third Report of the Dublin Hospital Initiative Group*, Dublin 1991

——, *Casemix Manual*, Dublin 1993

——, *Kilkenny Incest Investigation*, Dublin 1993

——, *Nursing Home Act*, Dublin 1994

——, *Shaping a Healthier Future: A Strategy for Effective Healthcare in the 1990s*, Dublin 1994

——, *White Paper: A New Mental Health Act*, Dublin 1995

——, *A Health Promotion Strategy*, Dublin 1995

——, *National Alcohol Policy*, Dublin 1996 (1996a)

——, *Report of Task Force on Travellers*, Dublin 1996 (1996b)

——, *National Task Force on Suicide: Interim Report*, 1996 (1996c)

——, *Putting Children First: a discussion document on mandatory reporting; Putting Children First: promoting and protecting the rights of children*, 1996 and 1997

Department of Health (UK), *The Health of the Nation (White Paper)*, HMSO 1992

Dineén, B. and Kelleher, C., 'Survey on Health Education and Health Promotion Activities by Relevant Organisations in Ireland', *Irish Educational Studies* 1995, 15: 183–193

Donabedian, A., *Explorations in Quality Assessment and Monitoring, Vol. I: The definition of quality and approaches to its assessment*, Ann Arbor, Michigan: Health Admin Pr 1980

——, *Explorations in Quality Assessment and Monitoring, Vol. II: The criteria and standards of quality*, Ann Arbor, Michigan: Health Admin Pr 1982

——., *Explorations in Quality Assessment and Monitoring, Vol. III: The methods and findings of quality assessment and monitoring, an illustrated analysis*, Ann Arbor, Michigan: Health Admin Pr 1985

Donnelly, M., 'Capacity of minors to consent to medical and contraceptive treatment', *Medico-Legal Journal of Ireland* 1995, 1 (1): 18–21

——, 'Confusion and uncertainty: the Irish approach to the duty to disclose risks in medical treatment', *Medico-Legal Journal of Ireland* 1996, 2 (1): 3

Doyle, Paddy, *The God Squad*, London 1989

Dublin Hospital Initiative Group, *Report*, Dublin 1991

Economic and Social Research Institute, *ESRI Medium-Term Review (1997–2003)*, Dublin 1997

Etzioni, Amitai, *The Spirit of Community*, London 1993

Evers, A., 'Welfare Pluralism and Personal Social Services: Analytical Concepts and Policy Developments', paper presented at COST conference, *Negotiated Economic and Social Governance and European Integration*, Dublin 1996

Eysenck, H.J., 'The Effects of Psychotherapy. An Evaluation', *J. Cons. Psychol.* 1952, XVI: 319–324

Fahey, T., Murray, P. and Whelan, B.J., *Health and Autonomy among the Over-65s in Ireland*, ESRI, Dublin 1993

Farmar, Tony, *Holles Street*, Dublin 1996

Farrar, S., 'NHS Reforms and Resource Management: Whither the Hospital?', *Health Policy* 1993, 26 (2): 93–104

Faughnan, P. and Healy, M., *Building Voluntary Sector Capacity*, action research programme on training needs in voluntary organisations, Social Science Research Centre, UCD 1997

Faughnan, P. and Kelleher, P., *The Voluntary Sector and the State*, Conference of Major Religious Superiors, Dublin 1992

Ferguson, Harry, 'Protecting Irish Children in Time: Child Abuse as a Social Problem and the Development of the Child Protection System in the Republic of Ireland', *Administration* 1996, 44 (2): 5–36

Fleetwood, J., *The History of Medicine in Dublin*, Dublin 1983

Food Safety Advisory Committee, *Diet and Cancer*, Dublin 1994

Frazer, Hugh, 'A Voice for the Voluntary and Community Sector', *Poverty Today* 1993 (July/Sept): 3

Gaskin, K. and Davis Smith, J., *A New Civic Europe? A study of the extent and role of volunteering*, London 1995

Giddens, A., *Modernity and Self-Identity*, Cambridge 1991

Gilligan, Robbie, *Irish Child Care Services – Policy, Practice and Provision*,

Dublin 1992

Goldbeck-Wood, S., 'Europe is divided on embryo regulations', *British Medical Journal* 1996, 313 (7056): 512

Graham, I. and Meleady, R., 'Heart Attacks and Homocysteine', *British Medical Journal* 1996, 313: 1419–20

Gunne, D. and O'Sullivan, B., 'Constructivist Psychotherapy', in Boyne (ed), *Psychotherapy in Ireland*, Dublin 1993

Guntz, H.P. and Guntz, S.P., 'Professional/Organisational Commitment and Job Satisfaction for Employed Managers', *Human Relations* 1994, 47 (7)

Haase, T. *et al.*, *Local Development Strategies for Disadvantaged Areas*, Area Development Management, Dublin 1996

Hannan, D. and O'Riain, S., *Pathways to Adulthood in Ireland*, Economic and Social Research Institute, Dublin 1993

Hanrahan, E. *Report on the Training of Student Nurses*, Irish Matrons' Association, Dublin 1975

Harding, S. and Balarjan, R., 'Patterns of mortality in second generation Irish living in England and Wales: longitudinal study', *British Medical Journal* 1996, 313: 1389–92

Harrigan, Mary Lou, *Quality of Care: Issues and Challenges in the 90s, a Literature Review*, Canadian Medical Association 1992

Hart, N., *The Sociology of Health and Medicine*, Ormskirk 1985

Harvey, B., *The National Lottery: Ten Years On*, Dublin 1995

——, *The Prospects for an Umbrella Organisation for the Voluntary Sector in Ireland*, Enterprise Trust, Dublin 1993

Hayes, T., *Management, Control and Accountability in Nonprofit/Voluntary Organizations*, Avebury 1996

Health Education Bureau, *Promoting Health through Public Policy*, Dublin 1987

Health and Safety Authority, *Guide to the Safety, Health and Welfare at Work Act 1989 and the Safety, Health and Welfare at Work (General Application) Regulations 1993*, Dublin 1995

Henry, H., *Our Lady's Psychiatric Hospital Cork*, Cork 1989

Hensey, Brendan, *The Health Services of Ireland*, Dublin 1988

Hickey, N. *et al.*, 'Study of coronary risk factors related to physical activity in 15,171 men', *British Medical Journal* 1975, 3: 507–10

Hogan, G., 'Wording to protect mother and foetus may never be found: conflicting definitions of abortion complicate search for legal solution', *Irish Times*, 4 March 1997

Hogan, G. and Whyte, G., *The Irish Constitution*, Dublin 1994

Hope, A. and Kelleher, C., *Health at Work*, Centre for Health Promotion Studies, Galway 1995

Inter-Departmental Committee on the Care of the Aged, *Report*, Dublin 1968

Inter Departmental Committee on the Reconstruction and Replacement of County Houses, *Report*, Dublin 1949

Irish Catholic Bishops' Advisory Committee on Child Sexual Abuse by Priests and Religious, *Report: Child Sexual Abuse: Framework for a Church Response*, Veritas 1996

Irish College of General Practitioners, *ICGP National Survey*, awaiting publication

Irish Council for Psychotherapy, *A Guide to Psychotherapy in Ireland*, Dublin 1997

Irish Health Research Board, *Activities of Irish Psychiatric Hospitals and Units 1991–1993*

Irish Heart Foundation, *Happy Heart National Survey, a report on Health Behaviour in Ireland*, 1994

Jacobs, K., 'The Management of Health Care: A Model of Control', *Health Policy* 1994, 19: 157–171

Joyce, P.W., *A Smaller Social History of Ancient Ireland*, London 1906

Keenan, O., *A Window on Irish Children*, unpublished paper presented to Barnardo's Annual Conference, 24 October 1991

Kelleher, Cecily, *Measures to Promote Health and Autonomy for Older People: a position paper*, National Council for the Elderly, Dublin 1993

Kelleher, P. and Whelan, M., *Dublin Communities in Action*, Dublin 1992

Kelly, F., *Window on a Catholic Parish*, Dublin 1996

Kennedy, S., *Who Should Care?*, Dublin 1981

Kennedy Report: *Report on the Reformatory and Industrial Schools System*, Committee on Reformatory and Industrial Schools, Dublin 1970

Kenny, V. (ed), 'Radical Constructivism, Antopoiesis and Psychotherapy', Special Edition, *Irish Journal of Psychology* 1984, 9 (1)

Keogh, F. and Walsh, D., *Irish Psychiatric Hospitals and Units: Activities 1995*, Health Research Board, Dublin 1996

Kickbusch, Ilona, 'New players for a new era: how up to date is health promotion?', *Health Promotion International* 1996, 11 (4): 259–261

Kramer, R., *Voluntary Agencies in the Welfare State*, California 1981

Kubler-Ross, E., *On Death and Dying*, Tavistock Publications 1979

Lacan, J., *Language of the Self*, Baltimore 1968

Law Commission, *The Law Commission: Mental Capacity*, Advance Statements about Health Care, Law Com. No. 231, HMSO 1995

Law Reform Commission, *Report on Personal Injury Awards*, 1997

Leff, J. *et al.*, 'A controlled trial of social intervention in families of schizophrenic patients', *British Journal of Psychiatry* 1982, 141: 121–134

McCarthy, G. *Student nurses in the Republic of Ireland: A study of their biographical, educational, motivational and personality characteristics*, MEd thesis, Trinity College Dublin, 1988

McCarthy, P. *et al.*, *Focus on Residential Child Care in Ireland: 25 years since the Kennedy Report*, FOCUS Ireland, Dublin 1996

McCashin, A., *Lone Mothers in Ireland*, Dublin 1996

McCluskey, D., *Health: People's Beliefs and Practices*, Dublin 1989

MacCulloch, M.J. and Feldman, P., 'Eye Movement Desensitisation Treatment Utilisation', *British Journal of Psychiatry* 1996, 169: 571–579

McGowan, J., *Attitude Survey on Irish Nurses*, Dublin 1979

McGuinness, C., *Report of the Kilkenny Incest Investigation*, Dublin 1993

McKeown, T. *The Modern Rise of Populations*, London 1976

McKevitt, David, *Health Care Policy in Ireland*, Hibernian University Press 1990

McLellan, T. *et al.* 'Are Psychosocial Services Necessary in Substance Abuse Treatment', *Journal of the American Medical Association* 1993 (April)

Madden, D., 'Medico-legal aspects of in vitro fertilisation and related infertility treatments', *Medico-Legal Journal of Ireland* 1995, 1 (1): 13–17

Magee, D., Browne, I. *et al.*, 'Unexperienced Experience: A critical reappraisal of the theory of repression', *Irish Journal of Psychology* 1984, 3: 7–11

Maggs, C., *The Origins of General Nursing*, London 1983

Mahon, E., 'From Democracy to Femocracy: The Women's Movement in the Republic of Ireland', in Clancy, P. *et al.* (eds), *Irish Society: Sociological Perspectives*, Dublin 1995

Mahon, E. and Conlon, C., 'Legal abortions carried out in England on women normally resident in the Republic of Ireland', Appendix 21, *Report of the Constitution Review Group*, Dublin 1996

Margison, Frank and McGrath, Graham, *Research in Psychotherapy, Research Methods in Psychiatry: A Beginner's Guide,* London, 105-119

Marinka Marshall Principles, *Medical Audit and General Practice*, London, 1990

Maturana, H. and Varela, F., *The Tree of Knowledge*, Shambala 1988

Mayer, P.G., 'Incorporating an Understanding of Independent Practice Physician Culture into Hospital Structure and Operations', *Hospital and Health Services Administration* 1992, 37 (4): 465–476

Medical Council, *A Guide to Ethical Conduct and Behaviour and to Fitness to Practice*, January 1994

Meehan, J., 'Principles for Partnership', *Poverty Today*, Combat Poverty Agency, Oct/Dec 1992: 7

Moller-Jensen, O. *et al.*, 'Cancer in the European Community and its member states', *European Journal of Cancer*, 26: 1167–1256

Murphy, Anne, *Attitudes of older people to heterodox and alternative health care systems*, PhD dissertation, in preparation, University College Galway

Murphy, Elaine, 'Meeting the needs of the most vulnerable', in Beck, E.J. and Adam, S. (eds), *The White Paper and Beyond*, Oxford Medical Publications 1990

National Council for the Aged, *Incomes of the Elderly in Ireland*, Dublin 1984

National Council for the Aged, *Caring for the Elderly*, Dublin 1988

National Economic and Social Council (NESC), *Health Services: The Implications of Demographic Change*, Dublin 1983

——, *Community Care Services: An Overview*, Dublin 1988

National Economic and Social Forum, *First Periodic Report on the Work of the Forum*, Forum Report No. 8, Dublin 1995

——, *Quality Delivery of Social Services*, Forum Report No. 6, Dublin 1995

National Nutritional Surveillance Centre, *Nutritional Surveillance in Ireland, 1993*, Centre for Health Promotion Studies, Galway 1993

National Social Services Board (NSSB), *The Development of Voluntary Social Services in Ireland: A Discussion Document*, Dublin 1982

National Social Services Board Strategy 1996–1998, NSSB 1996

Neate, J., *Quality Through Volunteers*, Volunteer Centre, UK 1996

Nedwick, N., 'Rights to NHS resources after the 1990 Act', *Medical Law Review* 1993, 1: 53–82

Nevis, E.C., 'Understanding Organisations and Learning Systems', *Sloan Management Review*, 1995 (winter): 73–85

Nic Gabhainn, S. and Kelleher, C., *Lifeskills for Health Promotion*, Centre for Health Promotion Studies, Galway 1995

——, *Attitudes of different socio-demographic groups to risk factors for cardiovascular disease*, submitted to Health Promotion Unit, Dept of Health, September 1996

Nightingale, F., *Notes on Nursing*, London 1952

Nolan, B., *et al.*, *Health Services Utilisation and Financing in Ireland*, ESRI Paper No. 155, Dublin 1991

Nutrition Advisory Group to Minister for Health, *Recommendations on a National Food Policy for Ireland*, Dublin 1995

O'Brien, T., 'Supreme Court decision in respect of a Ward of Court', *Irish Medical Journal* 1995, 88 (6): 183–187

O'Connor, J., *The Workhouses of Ireland*, Dublin 1995

O'Connor, P., 'Organisational Culture as a Barrier to Women's Promotion', *Economic and Social Review* 1996, 27 (3), 205–234

O'Donnell, R. and O'Reardon, C., 'Ireland's Experiment in Social Partnership 1987–1996', paper presented at COST conference, *Negotiated Economic and Social Governance and European Integration*, Dublin 1996

O'Donovan, Orla, *et al.*, *Advisory Report on a National Training Initiative for*

Formal Social Care Workers and Informal Carers of Older People, National Council for the Elderly, Dublin 1997

O'Donovan, O. and Casey, D., 'Converting Patients into Consumers: Consumerism and the Charter of Rights for Hospital Patients', *Irish Journal of Sociology* 1995, 5: 43–66

O'Dwyer, J. 'Nurse Education for the Future', paper presented at AGM of Irish Nurses' Organisation, 2 November 1984

OECD, *The Reform of Health Care: A Comparative Analysis of Seven OECD Countries*, Paris 1992

O'Neill, A.-M., 'Matters of discretion – the parameters of doctor/patient confidentiality', *Medico-Legal Journal of Ireland* 1995, 1 (3): 94–104

O'Sullivan, T., *A Service Without Walls*, Dublin 1995

O'Toole, Fintan, 'How Medical Council decided to admonish Ivor Browne', *Irish Times* 11 January 1997, 17

Outline of Proposals for the Improvement of the Health Services, Stationery Office, Dublin 1947

Phelan, D. and Kinirons, B., 'Withdrawal of futile interventions in intensive care – an everyday ethical/critical care issue', *Medico-Legal Journal of Ireland* 1996, 2 (2): 49–51

Phillips, A. *et al.*, 'Life Expectancy in men who have never smoked and those who smoked continuously: 15-year follow up of large cohort of middle-aged British men', *British Medical Journal* 1996, 313: 907–8

Podvoll, E., *The Seduction of Madness*, Harper Perennial 1990

Powell, F. 'Surveillance and Segregation: The Foundations of Irish Health Policy', *Administration*, 37 (1): 63–86

Pyle, J., *The State and Women in the Economy: Lessons from Sex Discrimination in the Republic of Ireland*, New York 1990

Rafferty, Mary, *Consultation, a Working Paper prepared for the Commission on the Status of People with Disabilities*, 1996

Report on the Training and Employment of the Handicapped, Stationery Office, Dublin 1974

Review Committee on the Adoption Service, *Report*, May 1984 (P1 2467)

Robbins, D., 'The Core of the Community', paper prepared for *Partners in Progress: The Role of NGO's* (conference, Galway), Dublin 1990

Robins, J., *The Lost Children: A Study of Charity Children in Ireland 1700–1900*, Dublin 1980

Rogers, C.R., *Client-Centered Therapy – Its Current Practice, Implications and Theory*, Boston 1951

Rose, Geoffrey, 'Sick Individuals and Sick Populations', *International Journal of Epidemiology* 1985, 14: 32–38

Ruddle, H. and Donoghue, F., *The Organisation of Volunteering*, Dublin 1995

Ruddle, H. and Mulvihill, R., *Reaching Out: Charitable Giving and Volunteering in the Republic of Ireland*, Dublin 1995

Sackett, D.L. *et al.*, *Clinical Epidemiology*, London 1991

———., 'Evidence based medicine: what it is and what it isn't', *British Medical Journal* 1996, 312: 71–2

Scanlon, P., *The Irish Nurse. A Study of Nursing in Ireland: History and Education 1718–1981*, Roscommon 1991

Shelley, E. *et al.*, 'Cardiovascular risk factor changes in the Kilkenny Health Project: A community health promotion programme', *European Heart Journal* 1995, 16: 752–60

Sixsmith, J., *Irish Women's Attitudes to Breast Cancer and Mammography: an urban-rural comparison*, Thesis for MA in Health Promotion, University College Galway 1995

Sixsmith, J. and Kelleher, C., *Evaluation of the Health Promotion Unit's Anti-Smoking Campaign 1996: 'Say what you like, smoking kills'. Stage I: National poll on campaign impact*, 1996 (unpublished)

Skrabanek, P. and McCormack, J., *Follies and Fallacies in Medicine*, Glasgow 1989

Smith, B. Abel, *A History of the Nursing Profession*, London 1980

Smith, M.L. and Glass, G.V., 'Meta-Analysis of Psychotherapy Outcome Studies', *Amer. Psych.* 1977, 32: 752–760

Smith, Richard, 'News: Gap between death rates of rich and poor widens', *British Medical Journal* 1997, 314: 9

Southgate, L. 'Freedom and Discipline: Clinical Practice and The Assessment of Clinical Competence', *British Journal of General Practice,* 44: 87-92

Spellman, J. see under Webb, M.

Stephens, Fred, *et al.*, 'Organisational and Professional Predictors of Physician Satisfaction', *Organisation Studies* 1992, 31 (1): 35–49

Stott, N.C.H. *et al.*, 'The Exceptional Potential in each Primary Care Consultation', *Journal of the Royal College of General Practitioners* 1979, 29: 201–205

Sutherland, Ralph W., *Health Care in Canada*, Canadian Public Health Association, Ottawa 1988

Task Force on Child Care Services, *Final Report*, Dublin 1981

The Years Ahead: A Policy for the Elderly, Stationery Office, Dublin 1988

Thorogood, M. *et al.*, 'Dietary intake and plasma lipid levels: lessons from a study of the diet of health conscious groups', *British Medical Journal* 1990, 300: 1297–1310

Tomkin, D. and Hanafin, P., 'Medical treatment at life's end: the need for legislation', *Medico-Legal Journal of Ireland* 1995, 1 (1): 3–10

Towards a Full Life: Green Paper on Services for Disabled People, Dublin 1989

Treacy, M., *In the pipeline: a qualitative study of General Nurse training with special reference to nurses' role in health education*, PhD thesis, University of London 1987

Tuairim Report, *Some of our Children – a report on the residential care of deprived children in Ireland*, London 1966

Tubridy, Jean, *Pegged Down*, Dublin 1996

Tussing, A. Dale, *Irish Medical Care Resources: An Economic Analysis*, ESRI Paper 126, Dublin 1985

Waldron, G. 'Crisis Intervention, is it effective?', *British Journal of Hospital Medicine* 1984 (April)

Warnock Commission, *Report of the Committee of Inquiry into Fertilisation and Embryology*, HMSO 1984

Webb, M., 'A psychiatrist's comments on the White Paper on a new mental health act'; Spellman, J., 'A lawyer's comments on the White Paper on a new mental health act', *Medico-Legal Journal of Ireland* 1995, 1 (3): 83–90

White, J., *Medical Negligence Actions*, Dublin 1996

White, K.L. *et al.*, 'The Ecology of Medical Care', *New Medical Journal of Medicine* 1961, 265: 885

Wiley, M., 'Budgeting for acute hospital services in Ireland: the case-mix adjustment', *Journal of the Irish Colleges of Physicians and Surgeons* 1995, 24 (4)

Wiley, M. and Fetter, R., *Measuring Activity and Costs in Irish Hospitals: A Study of Hospital Case Mix*, Dublin 1990

Willet, W.C. *et al.*, 'Dietary fat and the risk of breast cancer', *New England Journal of Medicine*, 316: 22–28

Wise, J., 'Storage period ends for 4000 embryos', *British Medical Journal*, 1996, 313 (7051): 189

World Health Authority (WHO), *Draft Charter of General Practice*, personal communication, awaiting publication, Copenhagen

Yalom, I., *Existential Psychotherapy*, New York 1980